JAMESTOW

THE
CONTEMPORARY
READER

VOLUME 2, NUMBER 6

ACKNOWLEDGEMENT
"Works from the Heart" adapted from "The Art and Heart of Horace Pippin" by Stephen May, *Smithsonian*, June 1994. Adapted with permission of author.

ISBN: 0-89061-831-3

Published by Jamestown Publishers,
a division of NTC/Contemporary Publishing Group, Inc.
4255 West Touhy Avenue,
Lincolnwood (Chicago), Illinois, 60712-1975, U.S.A.
© 1998 NTC/Contemporary Publishing Group, Inc..

01 02 03 04 WKT 10 9 8 7 6 5 4

CONTENTS

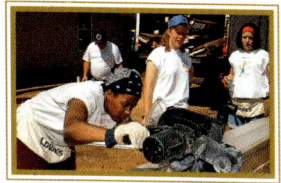

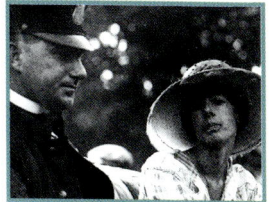

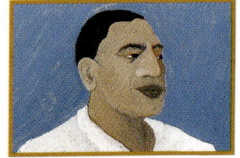

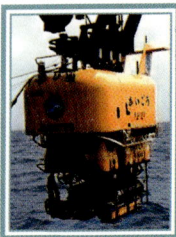

Pronunciation Key

ă	mat	o͞o	food
ā	date	o͝o	look
â	bare	ŭ	drum
ä	father	yo͞o	cute
ĕ	wet	û	fur
ē	see	*th*	then
ĭ	tip	th	thin
ī	ice	hw	which
î	pierce	zh	usual
ŏ	hot	ə	alone
ō	no		open
ô	law		pencil
oi	boil		lemon
ou	loud		campus

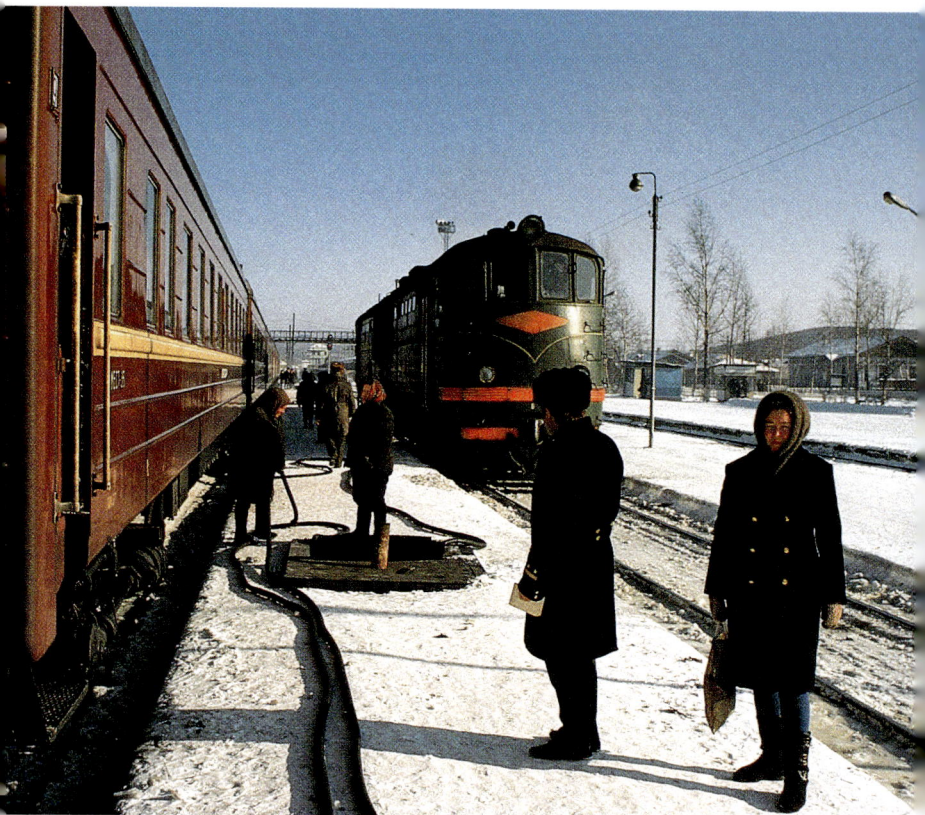

Linking Siberia with European Russia, the Trans-Siberian Railway has been a great boon to Russia's development.

THE WORLD'S LONGEST RAILWAY

What region of the world takes more than a week to cross by train?

1   In 1863, the United States began work on a transcontinental[1] railroad. Rails already ran from the East Coast to Omaha [ō′mə hô], Nebraska. The new track would extend from Omaha to California. In 1869, six years later, the monumental[2] task was completed. The workers had to cope with huge mountains, deep canyons, and miles of desert. The track ran halfway across the country.

2   As great as that project was, the Russians tried something even greater. They wanted to build a railroad across Siberia[3] [sī bîr′ē ə]. The entire

---

[1] transcontinental: crossing from one side of a land mass to another
[2] monumental: large and long-lasting
[3] Siberia: the northeastern region of Russia

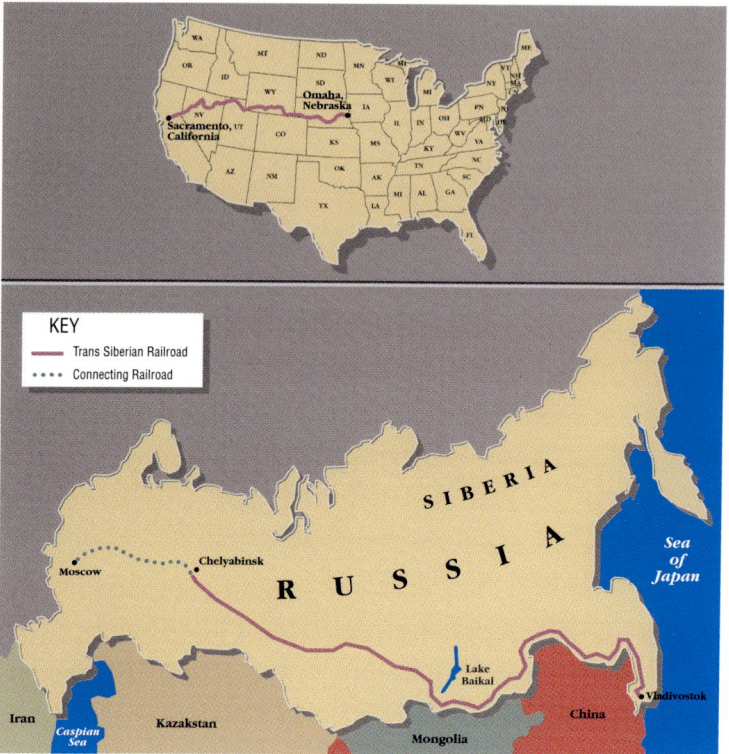

This map shows what a huge project the Trans-Siberian Railway was. Covering over 4,600 miles, the track length is more than three times that of the United States transcontinental railroad.

United States could fit inside Siberia, with 1.4 million square miles left over. Imagine the task of building a railroad across that distance!

A Grand Plan

3   The railroad was the grand dream of Czar [zär] Alexander III, the emperor of Russia. He needed the railroad to tie his vast land together. So, in 1891, as Alexander III laid the first stone, work began. The project called for two work crews.

One crew headed east and the other crew, west. Starting from opposite coasts and working inward, the two work crews planned to meet at a point in the middle.

4   Plans called for the track to run from Chelyabinsk [chĭ lyä′bĭnsk] in the west to Vladivostok [vlăd ə vŏs′tŏk] in the east, near the pacific coast. That distance would make the railroad the longest in the world—by far! It would cover 4,607 miles. The United States railroad was less than a third of that length.

5   Immigrant Irish and Chinese workers built the United States railroad. But the Russians used mostly convicts[4] and exiles[5] to build theirs. The poor job these men did would cause trouble with derailments[6] in the future.

Working Conditions

6   As it was, the railroad workers faced many problems. They had to cross wide rivers and climb steep grades.[7] In some places, the workers had to dig through permafrost. Permafrost, found just below the surface in frigid lands, is a layer of dirt that is frozen year round.

---

[4] convict: a prisoner
[5] exile: a person who has left or has been sent away from his or her country
[6] derailment: the result of a train running off the rails
[7] grade: a slope

7   Siberia is well known for its cold winters. This region has some of the lowest temperatures in the world. Forty degrees below zero Fahrenheit is common. At times, the air dips to 60 degrees below zero. Siberia's summers are not easy either. They can be brutally hot, with temperatures often soaring above 100 degrees. Even springtime, bringing ankle-deep mud, can be a problem.

8   Many workers died building this railroad. The work itself killed some of them. The harsh weather killed others. As if that weren't bad enough, a few other workers fell prey to Siberian tigers.

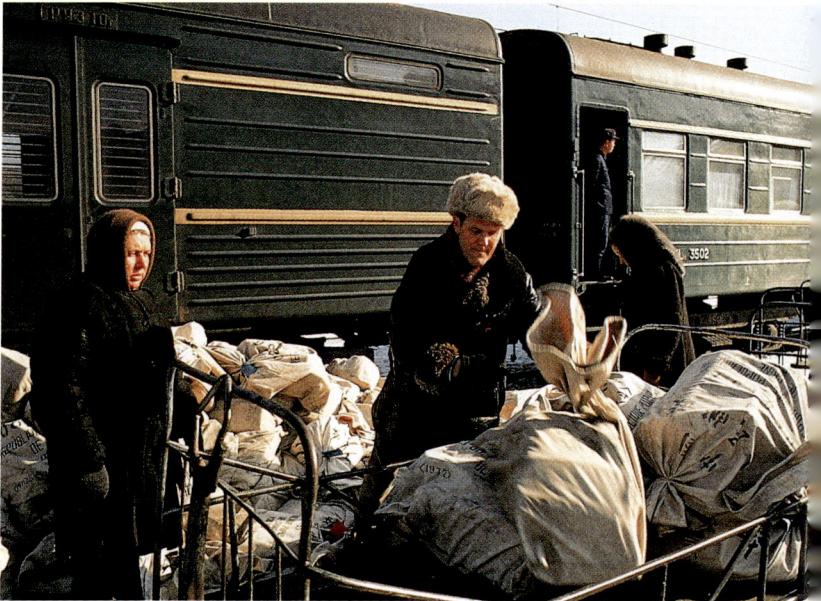

The sameness of the Siberian landscape can make loading the baggage the most interesting thing to see during the long train trip.

Political Problems

9   Nature was not the only hurdle in building the railroad. Politics caused trouble too. At first, the Russians wanted a route that passed through Russian land only. But in 1896, they signed a treaty with China. One outcome of the treaty shortened the route of the railroad. Part of the track would cut through the north of China.

10   Then, in 1904, war broke out between Russia and Japan. The fighting ended a year later when the Japanese crushed the Russians. Japan also took over the northern part of China. The Russians lost control of that land and the tracks that ran through it. So the Russian railroad would not cut through China, after all. The Russians returned to the old plan for an all-Russian route. At last, in 1917, the railroad was finished. It had taken more than 25 years to build.

Riding the Rails

11   The railroad opened before it was finished. By the end of 1900, trains began to make trips. But there were problems all along the way. Steep grades near the southern shore of Lake Baikal [bī kôl′] made it hard to lay tracks in that region. So passengers had to get off the train and cross the lake by ferryboat. In the end, the Russians had to build 38 tunnels through the mountains.

12   The biggest problems, however, were derailments. The trains couldn't be trusted to stay

on the tracks. On an average trip, a train would jump the tracks twice. Operators at the time had the good sense to run the trains slowly. The average top speed was just 15 miles per hour. At that slow speed, a derailment didn't often hurt people. But the snail-like pace annoyed travelers. If all went well, a trip across the continent was supposed to take two weeks. Instead, the trip always took longer than three weeks to complete.

The Trans-Siberian Railroad Today

13   Through the years, the Russians improved the Trans-Siberian Railroad. A second set of tracks was laid by 1939 and is still in use today.

14   Now people can hop on a train in Moscow and ride it all the way east to the Sea of Japan. The railroad is, of course, much more reliable today than in the past. But even a smooth trip takes at least 170 hours—more than seven days—to complete.

15   For true railroad buffs,[8] riding the Trans-Siberian Railroad is a must. Most of these people take the trip just to say that they did it. Surely, no one takes the trip for the scenery. At least, no one takes it for the *variety* of scenery: Siberia is one vast, empty plain.[9] Whoever made up the phrase "the middle of nowhere" must have had Siberia in

[8] buff: a person who enjoys a subject and knows a lot about it

[9] plain: a large, flat, treeless area

mind. As one writer put it, there is "nothing but hut, tree, hut, filing by with the dull rhythm of a forced march."

16   Still, the railroad has played a vital role in the development of Russia. It has opened up Siberia to settlers. It has also helped industry, for Siberia is rich in natural resources. It has large amounts of oil, coal, natural gas, and iron. The railroad route has linked Siberia's mining centers with Russia's main business areas. Without the railroad, Siberia's natural riches would lie untouched and of little use.

17   The railroad has become a lifeline between Siberia and European Russia. This important outcome may have reached beyond even Czar Alexander's greatest dream.

QUESTIONS

1. Why did Czar Alexander want a Trans-Siberian railroad?
2. Name two ways in which building the Trans-Siberian Railroad was different from building the U.S. transcontinental railroad.
3. What dangers did the Russian railroad builders face?
4. Why is the trip across Siberia boring?
5. Why is the Trans-Siberian Railroad important to Russia today?

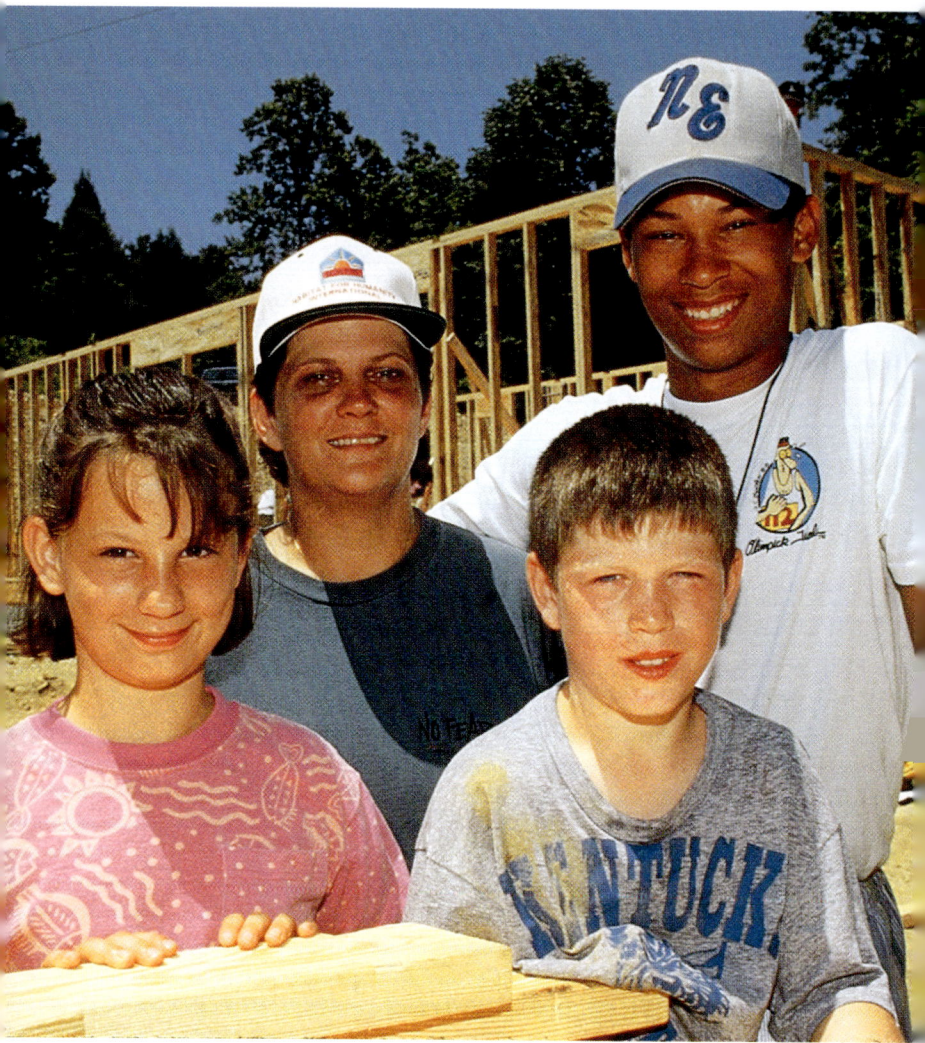

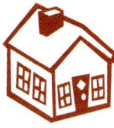

Habitat for Humanity

How does Habitat for Humanity help people in need?

1 A decent home. A safe neighborhood. An affordable mortgage. These have always been part of the American Dream. Yet for many families, this dream seems impossible. These are families in need who struggle to pay their bills and to save money. They cannot afford to buy a house.

2 Such families might lose hope. They may feel that the American Dream is out of reach or that it has passed them by.

A Helping Hand

3 For more than 20 years, a group has helped needy families reach this dream. The group is called Habitat for Humanity. Millard and Linda Fuller, a couple from Georgia, founded the group

Habitat for Humanity invites people from all walks of life to work together to build houses for families in need.

in 1976. Habitat for Humanity is a nonprofit[1]
group. It has one goal: to get rid of poverty-level
housing and homelessness around the world.

4   The goal is great. But Habitat for Humanity
moves toward it step by step. Since 1976, the
group has built or fixed up more than 50,000
homes. These homes shelter about 250,000
people around the world.

How It Works

5   As a nonprofit group, Habitat for Humanity relies
on gifts and volunteers. It seeks donations[2] of
money, land, and supplies. To keep building
costs low, the group tries to get as many gifts as
possible. In turn, the group can sell the homes at
a very low price. Habitat for Humanity passes the
savings on to home buyers. The average price for
a three-bedroom home is $38,000.

6   It takes hard work to get donations. Habitat
for Humanity tries to raise money through fund-
raisers.[3] Habitat workers ask cities and wealthy
landowners to donate land.

7   The group also seeks gifts from building
supply companies. It asks for any materials a
company can spare. For example, one company

---

[1] nonprofit: not for the purpose of making money
[2] donation: a gift of money or goods
[3] fundraiser: a social event held to raise money for a cause

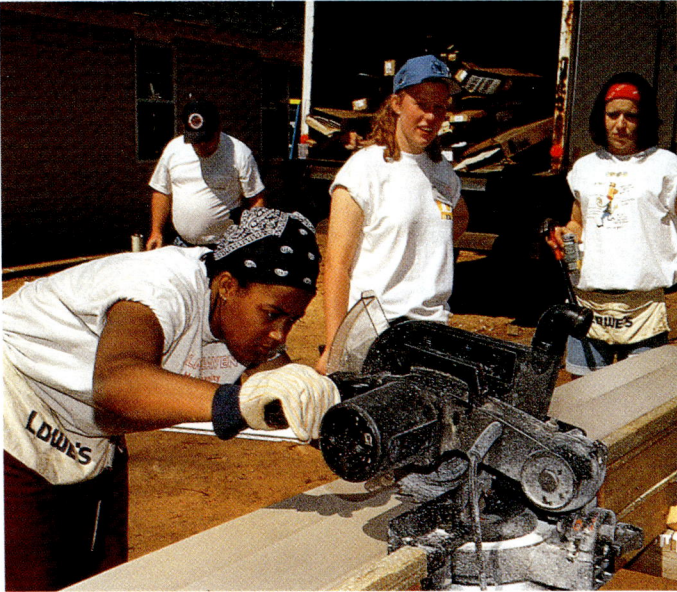

Volunteers work side by side with future homeowners, who become partners with Habitat for Humanity. Partner families put in about 500 hours of labor, or "sweat equity," to build their homes and the homes of others. Raising funds for Habitat and working in the Habitat offices also count as sweat equity hours.

might donate windows, carpeting, or paint. Another company might provide nails or tools.

8   Finally, the group must find volunteer builders. It needs skilled workers. But it uses unskilled workers too. Habitat trains workers on the job, so it welcomes anyone who will pick up a hammer.

The Homeowner's Role

9   Habitat for Humanity works hard to find just the right homeowners. The staff screens each person

who wants to buy a home. A family must meet several conditions to be a homeowner. The family must be needy, but it must have some income. Homeowners get an interest-free loan[4] from the Habitat group. They must be able to make monthly payments to pay back the loan in 20 years. These payments are used to fund other Habitat homes.

10   Homeowners also must be willing to work as partners with Habitat for Humanity. They put in their share of "sweat equity." In other words, they must pitch in and help the Habitat workers. Homeowners may help get donations, run the group office, or build homes. Each owner must put in about 500 hours of sweat equity.

11   Albertha Whiteside bought a Habitat home in 1993. As part of her sweat equity, she answered Habitat's phones and sent out newsletters. She also helped frame and hang drywall in her new house. "This is where I learned to pound my first nail," she says with pride.

12   Habitat for Humanity is not a giveaway program. It is a partnership. Habitat becomes a partner with the homeowner. The result is decent housing that is safe and affordable.

---

[4] interest-free loan: a loan that does not require payment of an added fee for use

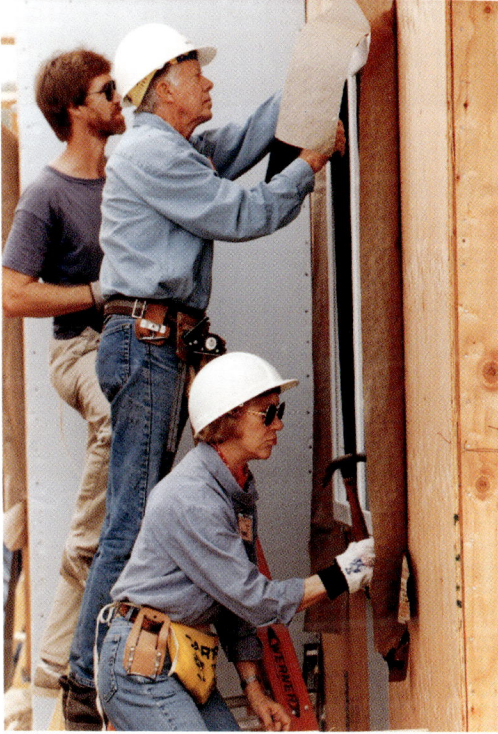

Former President Jimmy Carter and his wife, Rosalyn, pitch in to build a Habitat house near Los Angeles, California. The Carters have worked with Habitat for Humanity since 1980 and still give "hands-on" support to housing programs.

Happy Endings

13 The partnership has other results. One example is the chance for buyers to learn useful home management skills. The Habitat program offers workshops for buyers. In them, buyers learn to maintain their homes and to budget their money.

14   Perhaps the best result is the program's effect on families. Buyers say that home ownership greatly improves their lives. Whiteside says that living in the new home has changed her family. Her children are happier, and her marriage has improved. She feels better about herself too. "I've always been a positive person," she said. "But I'm much happier and more relaxed now."

15   Whiteside also notes a big difference between renting and owning. Owning has taught her to budget and save. For minor repairs, Whiteside now depends on herself instead of a landlord. "I'm more mature, more responsible, and more independent," she says.

16   Rená Bligen agrees. "Habitat was the answer to our prayers," she says. Countless others are quick to praise the Habitat program.

A Worldwide Program

17   Habitat for Humanity began as a small group but grew quickly. It now has 1,300 branches in the United States, with branches in all 50 states. The program's 250 more branches around the world build houses in more than 50 nations.

18   The program got an unexpected boost in the 1980s. President Jimmy Carter ran for reelection in 1980, but he lost. After this defeat, he and Mrs. Carter joined Habitat for Humanity. His work helped promote the program. Because of

the Carters, the program became better known, and many people joined it.

19   The Fullers founded Habitat as a Christian ministry.[5] It still has a Christian focus. In some ways, however, it cuts across the boundaries of religion. "Over the last 20 years, it has really spread out across church lines," says one Habitat director. "There are many people [involved with Habitat] who have no affiliation[6] to a particular church. These are people who still want to find ways to help their fellow human beings."

Q U E S T I O N S

1. What is the goal of Habitat for Humanity?

2. How does Habitat for Humanity keep the cost of its houses down?

3. What does Habitat for Humanity require of home buyers?

4. List two ways in which Habitat for Humanity changed homeowners' lives.

5. What famous Americans are involved with Habitat for Humanity?

---

[5] ministry: a service or duty
[6] affiliation: a link or connection

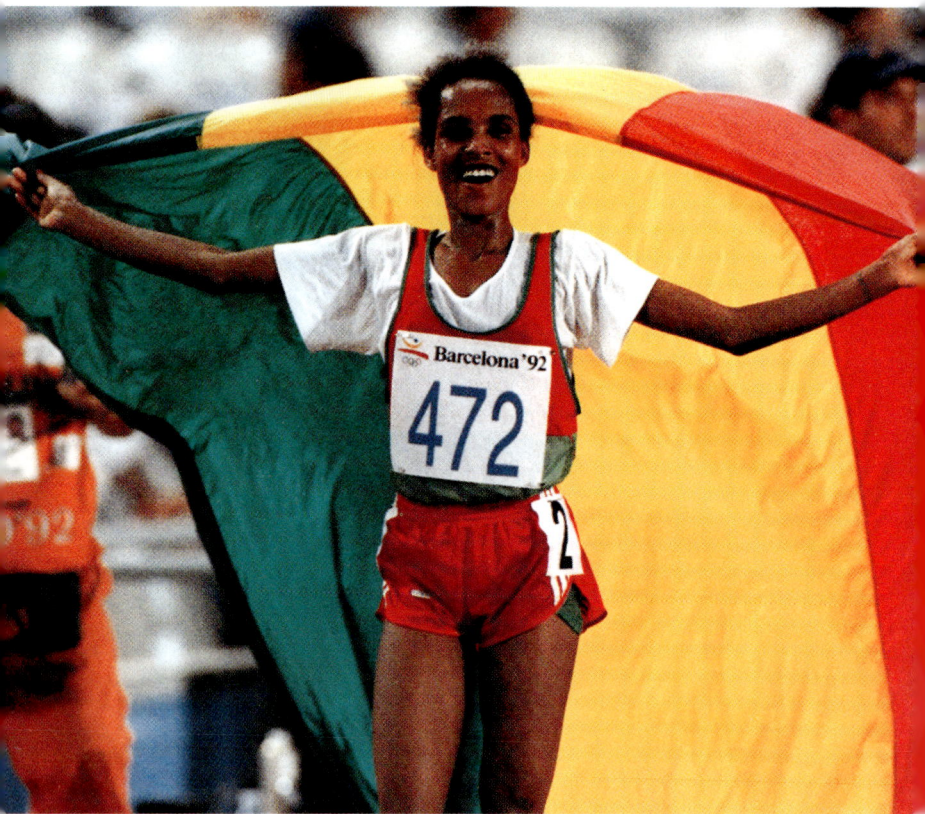

Runner Derartu Tulu of Ethiopia, a country in Africa, waves a giant national flag after her victory. She won the women's 10,000-meter race at the 1992 Summer Olympics in Spain.

THE **BIRTH** OF THE **MODERN OLYMPICS**

Why were the Olympic Games revived?

1   The first official Olympic Games took place in Olympia, Greece, in 776 B.C. Some games were held to honor the gods. Others were offerings of thanksgiving. The games were held for hundreds of years. They went on even after the Romans took over Greece in A.D.146. When the games first began, the athletes were amateurs[1] [ăm´ ə tûrz]. But as time passed, the games grew more professional. Athletes began to compete for personal glory. Many winners put up statues to honor themselves. The original purpose of the games had become lost.

2   As a result, the public grew disgusted and lost interest in the games. In A.D. 394, the games finally came to an end. A Roman emperor outlawed them. The Olympics, said the ruler, had become corrupt.

---

[1] amateur: an athlete who does not compete for money or to earn a living

Pierre de Coubertin

3   For 1,500 years the games remained dead. But
thanks to one man from France, they came back
to life. The man's name was Baron Pierre de
Coubertin [pyâr də kōō bâr tăn′]. He wanted
very much to revive the ancient Olympics.
However, he thought the Olympics should be
more than just fun and games. They should
fulfill[2] a higher purpose.

4   De Coubertin wanted the games to promote
peace among nations. "Sport is not a luxury," he
said. "It is a necessity. Let us bring the nations
together for friendly [games]. . . ."

5   De Coubertin felt that the games should serve
to teach the young. Like the Greeks of old, he
knew the importance of balancing the growth of
both mind *and* body. De Coubertin also hoped
that the Olympics would inspire the young. The
goal of the games, he said, was "to create a way
of life based on the joy of effort."

6   De Coubertin believed in fair play and in the
"spirit of competition." He once said, "The most
important thing is not to win, but to take part."
He compared this idea to life. "[It is] not the tri-
umph, but the struggle. The essential[3] thing is not
to have conquered, but to have fought well."

---

[2] fulfill: to satisfy
[3] essential: basic; needed

Selling His Ideas

7   Selling his idea for the modern Olympics wasn't easy. In 1892, de Coubertin began his tireless campaign [kăm pān′] to revive the games. At first, no one cared much. But de Coubertin would not give up.

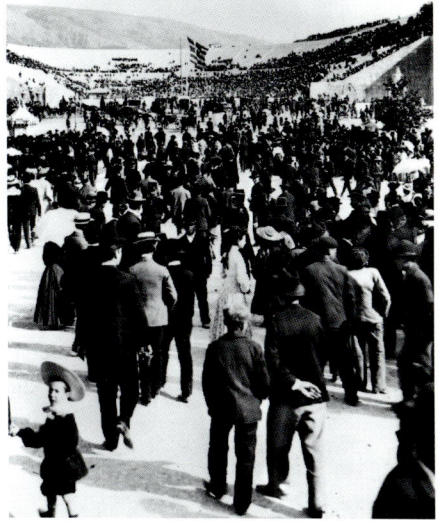

The 1896 Olympic Games, held in Athens, Greece, marked the birth of the modern Olympics. More than 60,000 fans crowded the stadium, a restored structure that dated from ancient times.

8   Two years later, in 1894, de Coubertin brought together 79 delegates[4] from 12 countries. They met to discuss a revival of the Olympic Games. After a passionate plea by de Coubertin, nine nations gave him their full support. The first modern games were set for 1896. The nations agreed that the games would be held every four years in great cities of the world.

9   De Coubertin wanted the first Olympics to be held in France. Others, however, felt that Greece was a better choice, since the Greeks had started the games. De Coubertin agreed, and in return, France hosted the second Olympics.

---

[4] delegate: a person who represents another person or group of people at a meeting

The IOC

10   When they had first met in 1894, the nine nations who voted to revive the games also set up the International Olympic Committee, or IOC. The IOC's purpose is to look after the growth and improvement of the Olympics. The members of the IOC were free from outside pressure. No nation could tell the committee how to run the Olympics.

11   De Coubertin thought the IOC's first president should be Greek. The man chosen was Demetrius Vikelas [də mē′trē əs vē′kə ləs],

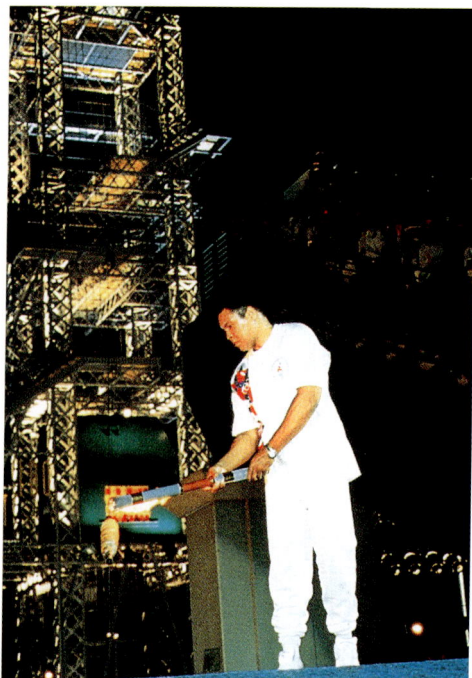

Muhammed Ali, former boxing champion and Olympic gold medalist, lights the flame to open the 1996 Olympics in Atlanta, Georgia.

who began his term in 1894. In 1896, de Coubertin took over the job and held it for 30 years.

The 1896 Olympics

12   The first modern Olympic Games, held in Athens, Greece, were a great success. King George I of Greece opened the games. More than 60,000 fans packed the stands on opening day.

13   Thirteen countries competed in the games. Only nine sports were involved. They included some of the original Olympic sports such as running and wrestling. But modern sports such as lawn tennis and cycling were also scheduled.

14   Francis Lane, an American, won the first event. He ran 100 meters in 12.5 seconds and won a silver medal for his skill. At that time, only one type of medal was awarded—a silver medal.

Olympic Customs

15   As president of the IOC, de Coubertin made changes to the Olympics that are still in use today. Starting with the 1908 games, the top *three* finishers got medals—gold, silver, and bronze. Both the five-ringed Olympic flag and the Olympic oath were first used in 1920.

16   In later years, the IOC added more customs. The lighting of the Olympic flame began with the 1928 games. So did the custom of releasing a flock of doves as a sign of hope for world peace.

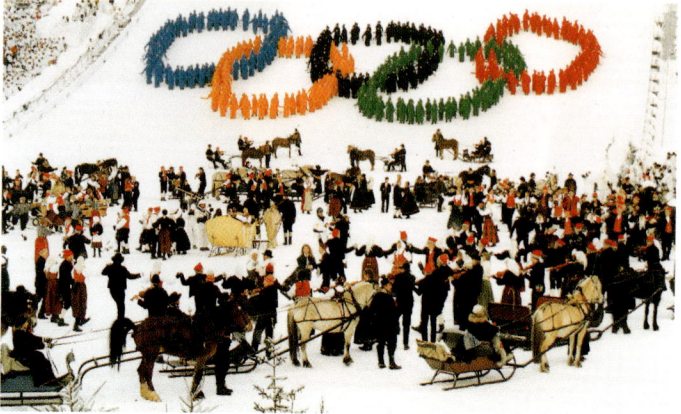

At the 1994 Olympics in Norway, performers themselves form the familiar five Olympic rings as folk dancers entertain the fans.

17   The first Winter Olympics were held in 1924. Since then, new winter and summer sports have been added to the games. The number of athletes who compete has shot up over time. In 1896, 311 men took part. Now thousands of athletes, both male and female, enter the games. Women first took part in the Olympics in 1900, playing lawn tennis. Today the Olympics involve almost all nations of the world. The games have grown in ways de Coubertin never dreamed of.

The Fate of de Coubertin's Ideals[5]

18   The old games died out when they grew too professional. De Coubertin did not want to see

5 ideal: a perfect model

them end once again. So for a long time, the modern games were open only to amateurs. Athletes took part for the love of sports. That ideal, however, is gone; the modern Olympics are now open to anyone. The U.S.A. basketball Dream Team (in 1992 and 1996), made up of professional athletes, was not what de Coubertin had in mind.

19   Other ideals have also fallen by the wayside. It no longer seems enough just to compete. Everyone wants to *win*. Fans love the winners and forget the losers. Sadly, the drive to win has corrupted the ideal of fair play. Some athletes have used drugs to increase their chances of winning. In spite of these lost ideals, however, the Olympic games remain as popular as ever.

20   De Coubertin died in 1937. His body is buried in Lausanne [lō zăn′], Switzerland, but his heart rests at Olympia, Greece.

QUESTIONS

1. Why did the first Olympic Games end?
2. Why did Pierre de Coubertin want to revive the games?
3. What ideals did Pierre de Coubertin want to promote?
4. What is the IOC?
5. What has happened to the ideals of Pierre de Coubertin?

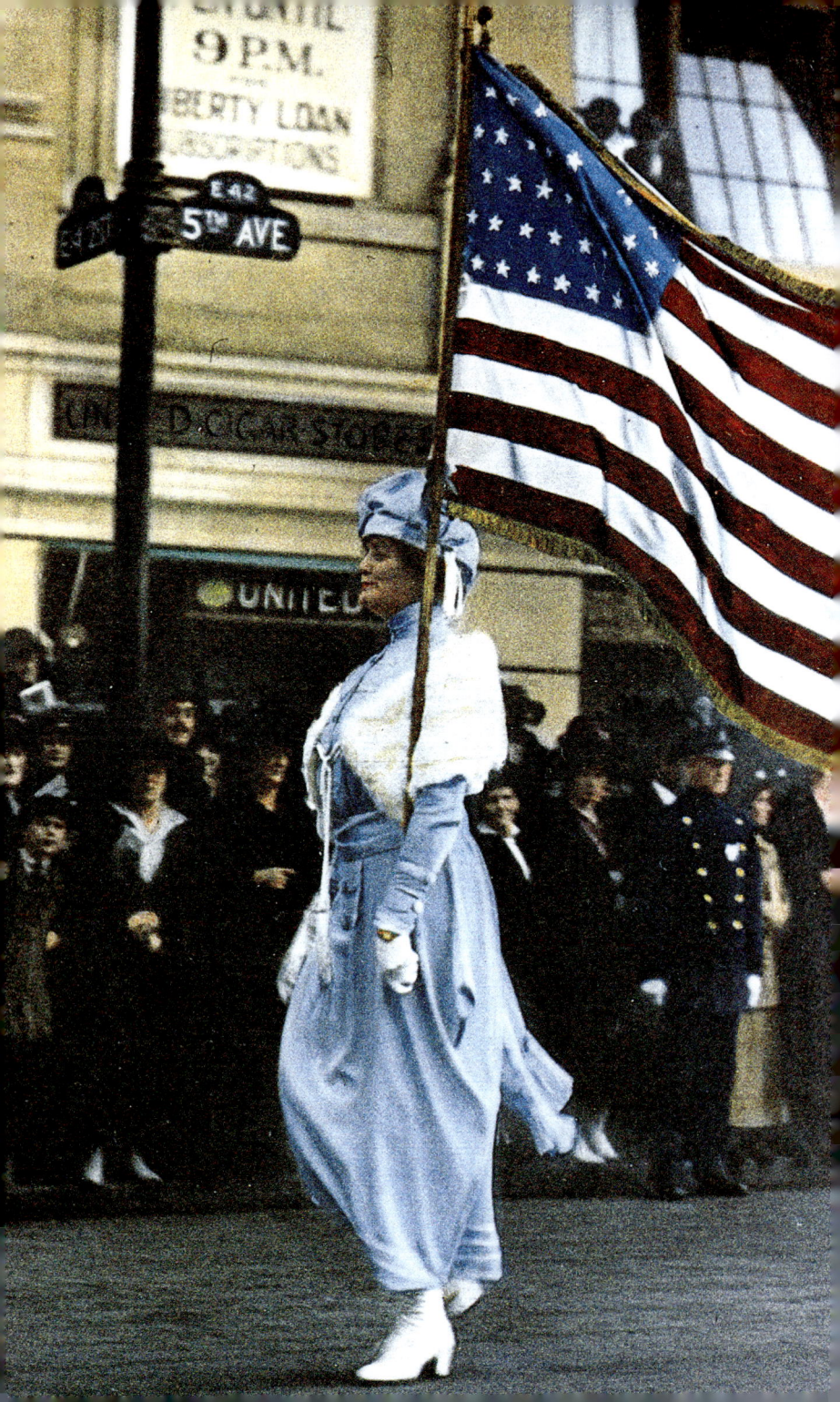

Battle *of the* Ballot

*How would you feel if you had lived at
a time when women couldn't vote?*

1 Picture yourself living in 1848. Women in the
United States aren't allowed to vote. They can't
own property. They can't serve on juries or even
go to most colleges!

2 Many women were upset about these things.
They knew that change had to come, and soon.
In 1848, about 300 women met in Seneca Falls,
New York, to hold the first Women's Rights
Convention.

3 At this meeting, the women talked about their
goals. They wanted to buy property in their own
names. Like men, they wanted the right to a
good education. Most important, they wanted the
right to vote. With the vote, they would be the
political equals of men.

**Bearing the American flag, a woman marches for the right
to vote. This struggle for political equality lasted more than
70 years.**

4   A few women were nervous about asking for the vote. They couldn't believe they would ever get it. But they decided to work for it anyway.

Banding Together

5   For many years, women had banded together to fight social problems. Many groups had spoken out against slavery. Others fought to ban alcoholic drinks or to improve education. Word spread about the brave women in Seneca Falls. Other groups joined the fight for women suffrage.[1] Many had gained skills from their group work. Now they used these skills to change the minds of the American public.

Two Leaders

6   Two women stand out as the leaders in the struggle for the right to vote. Neither lived to see the laws changed. But their hard work started the movement. These women refused to let the dream of equal rights die.

7   Elizabeth Cady Stanton was the mother of six children. She was an excellent writer and speaker. Her father had been a judge. As a child, Stanton saw how unfair the law was to women, and she vowed to change it.

---

[1] suffrage: the right to vote

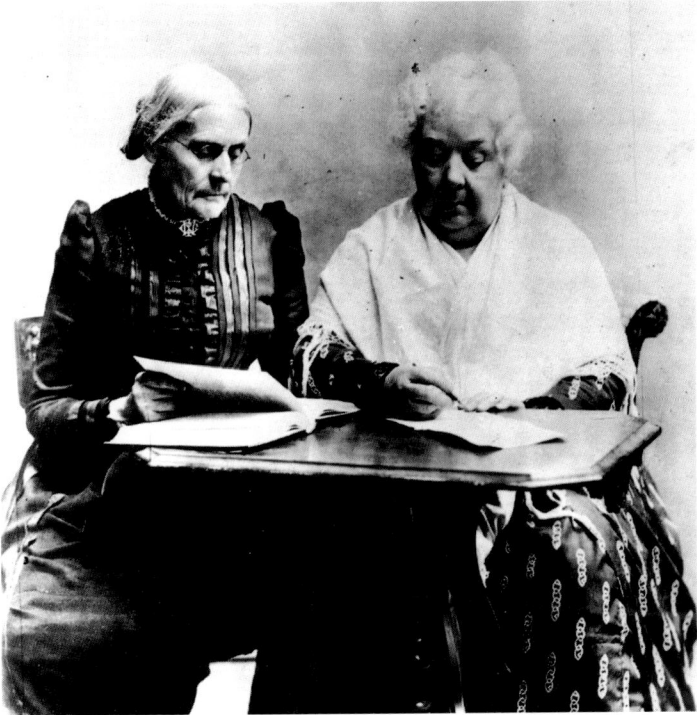

Susan B. Anthony (left) and Elizabeth Cady Stanton led the movement for women's suffrage. Their work kept alive the question "If women are citizens, why can't they vote?"

8   Mrs. Stanton's best friend was Susan B. Anthony. Anthony grew up in a Quaker family. She had been active in the fight against slavery. She had strong feelings about justice.

9   Anthony taught school for several years. One day, she learned that a male teacher was earning $40 a month while Anthony made only $10. The pay was different only because she was a woman. Her sense of justice told her to work for women's rights.

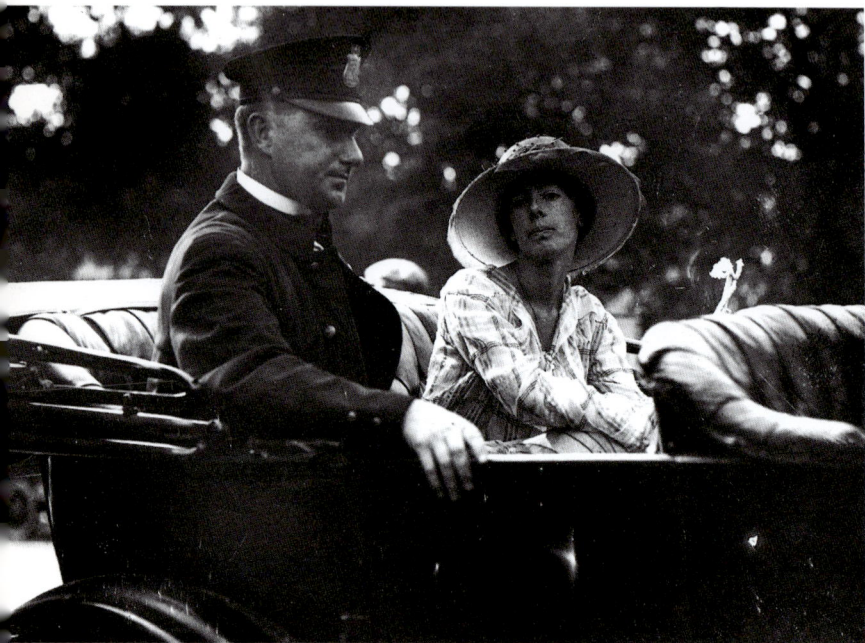

Before they had the right to vote, women who cast ballots were arrested for breaking the law. It doesn't look as if a trip to jail could discourage this suffragist's fight.

Call to Action

10   Anthony began to organize[2] women to try to change the law. She planned women's meetings and conventions. She gave speeches written by Stanton, who was often busy with her young children. Anthony felt that people needed to hear her words.

11   In 1869, Anthony and Stanton formed the National Woman Suffrage Association (NWSA).

---

[2] organize: to form a group with a specific purpose

The group's goal was an amendment[3] to the Federal Constitution that gave women the right to vote. That year another group formed called the American Woman Suffrage Association (AWSA). This group did not work toward one main law for women suffrage. Instead, the AWSA strove for a suffrage amendment to each state constitution.

12   Stanton, Anthony, and many other women spoke to groups of people all over the United States. They urged citizens to write to their leaders. They asked lawmakers to change the laws. They asked men as well as women to sign petitions.[4] The important question put to the public was "If women are citizens, why can't they vote?"

Not Always Welcome

13   Workers for women's rights were not always welcome in places where they gathered to speak. During speeches, people threw eggs and vegetables. They made fun of the women suffragists and called them names. Even many women slammed doors in their faces. Men laughed at what the suffragists said. Newspapers poked fun at the way they dressed. Little by little, however, people's minds began to change. But even after years of work, women still didn't have the right to vote.

---

[3] amendment: an addition or correction to a law
[4] petition: a formal written request to one who is above another in rank or office

14   In 1870, a new amendment to the Constitution granted the vote to male ex-slaves. The new law made the suffragists impatient [ĭm pā′shənt]. In 1872, some women decided to vote anyway. They felt that the new amendment was meant as much for women as for the male ex-slaves. Susan B. Anthony was among this group of women. On November 5, 1872, Anthony walked into a polling place[5] in Rochester, New York. She signed up to vote and demanded a ballot[6] from the election staff. She said that the Constitution gave all citizens the right to vote. Then she cast her ballot in the presidential election held that year.

15   Later, Anthony wrote these words to Stanton: "Well, I have been and gone and done it, positively voted this morning at 7 o'clock. . . . Now if all our suffrage women would work to this end . . . what strides we might make from now on!"

On Trial

16   Because she had broken the law, Anthony was arrested. She had to stand trial for voting. The judge found her guilty and fined her $100. Anthony said she would never pay the unjust fine. Even so, she was released.

---

[5] polling place: a location where registered citizens can cast a vote

[6] ballot: a sheet of paper used for voting

17   In 1875, the Supreme Court considered whether women had the right to vote. They said that the Constitution did *not* give women the right to vote. They *were* citizens, but not *all* citizens had the right to vote. The suffragists were disappointed, but they didn't give up. Now they knew they had to change the Constitution.

Two Groups Unite

18   In 1890, the two major women's rights groups (the NWSA and the AWSA) united. They formed

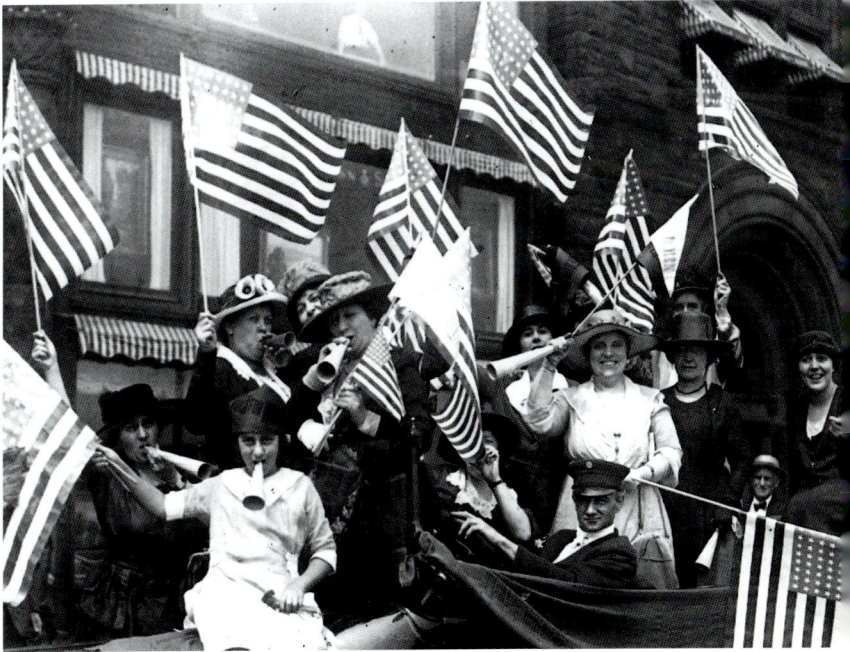

Suffragists celebrate their hard-won victory—the passage of the Nineteenth Amendment to the United States Constitution. The amendment, which allows all U.S. citizens to vote in elections, became law in 1920.

the National American Woman Suffrage
Association. For the next 29 years, this group
worked to change the Constitution.

19   Over and over, the suffragists sent congressmen copies of the "Anthony Amendment." This
amendment would give women the right to vote.
The suffragists urged people to write to their
congressmen. They stood outside the White
House, calling out to the president each time he
came or left. They marched in parades in cities
and towns across the country.

Success at Last

20   Finally, in 1919, Congress passed the Nineteenth
Amendment to the Constitution. This is how it
reads:

> The right of citizens of the United States
> to vote shall not be denied or abridged[7] by
> the United States or by any State on account
> of sex.

By the end of August 1920, two-thirds of the
states had approved the amendment. It became
the law of the land.

21   The election of November 1920 made history.
For the first time, and in every state, women were
allowed to cast votes. The right they had been
denied [dĭ nīd'] for so long was finally theirs.

------

[7] abridged: shortened

Questions

1. Which group met in Seneca Falls, New York, in 1848?
2. What was the most important thing the women wanted?
3. What happened to Susan B. Anthony after she voted in 1872?
4. When did Congress pass the Nineteenth Amendment?
5. State in your own words what the Nineteenth Amendment says.

MOUNT WASHINGTON
SMALL BUT DEADLY

Why is Mount Washington often called the most dangerous small mountain in the world?

1 Mount Washington, located in the state of New Hampshire, is 6,288 feet high. That height isn't too impressive: hundreds of mountains are much higher than that. Mount Whitney, in California, is more than twice as high. Mount McKinley, in Alaska, is more than three times as high. And Mount Everest, on the continent of Asia, is nearly five times as high.

2 Yet no one should take Mount Washington for granted. Those who do could pay a high price for their mistake. Well over 100 people have died on Mount Washington. The trails on the way up the mountain are dotted with little markers. These markers describe when and how a death occurred[1] at each spot.

---

[1] occurred: happened

The top of Mount Washington has perhaps the world's worst weather. High winds, raging blizzards, or a thick fog like this one have led to death for hikers and skiers caught off guard.

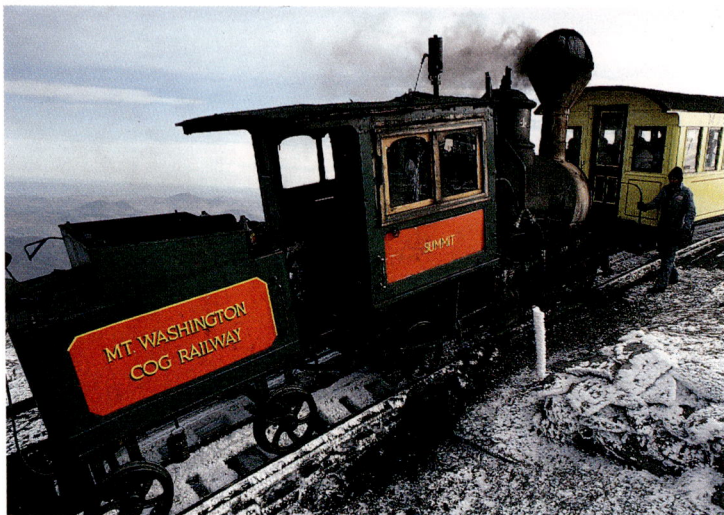

The 3-mile-long Cog Railway is one popular way to reach the top of Mount Washington. The tracks have the steepest slope of any in the United States.

The World's Worst Weather

3   Every so often, the weather is good at the top of Mount Washington. But sunshine can't be counted on. The weather is almost always nasty. In fact, many people in New Hampshire say that Mount Washington has the world's worst weather. Although that claim is open to debate, everyone agrees that the weather at the peak is nearly always awful.

4   A look at some of the numbers will show the reason. The highest wind speed ever recorded on Earth was on Mount Washington. It happened on April 12, 1934 when the wind gusted at 231 miles per hour!

5   On average, winds of hurricane force—or winds of more than 74 miles per hour—rise up every third day. Nature once piled 566 inches of snow on top of Mount Washington in one winter alone. In addition, it is almost always cold on the mountain. Below-zero temperatures are common. When the high winds are added to the bitter cold, the weather on Mount Washington rivals[2] that in Antarctica. When the wind finally dies down, a fog as thick as pea soup usually rolls in.

6   Even worse, the weather is not predictable. Things might look fine from the lodge[3] at the base of the mountain. But on top, the weather can change in the blink of an eye. That is why so many hikers—even hardy ones—die on the mountain. They are not prepared for the worst.

Weather Hazards

7   Mount Washington's top 1,500 feet or so lie above the timberline.[4] Once there, a person has no protection from the weather. A sudden storm can appear out of nowhere. Blinding snow and cold can easily kill people.

---

[2] rival: to be equal to or match
[3] lodge: a cabinlike hotel or inn
[4] timberline: the point on a mountainside beyond which trees do not grow

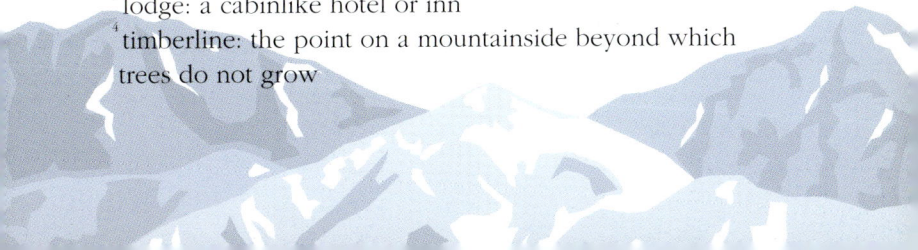

8   A driving mountain rain can kill people too. A cold summer rain may be the greatest danger of all, for rain soaks through clothing faster than snow does. When heat is drained from a person's body, the result is a condition called *hypothermia* [hī pō thûr′ mē ə]. As the body loses heat, the brain slows down. The person can no longer think clearly and becomes confused and dazed. He or she may fall down and never get up again.

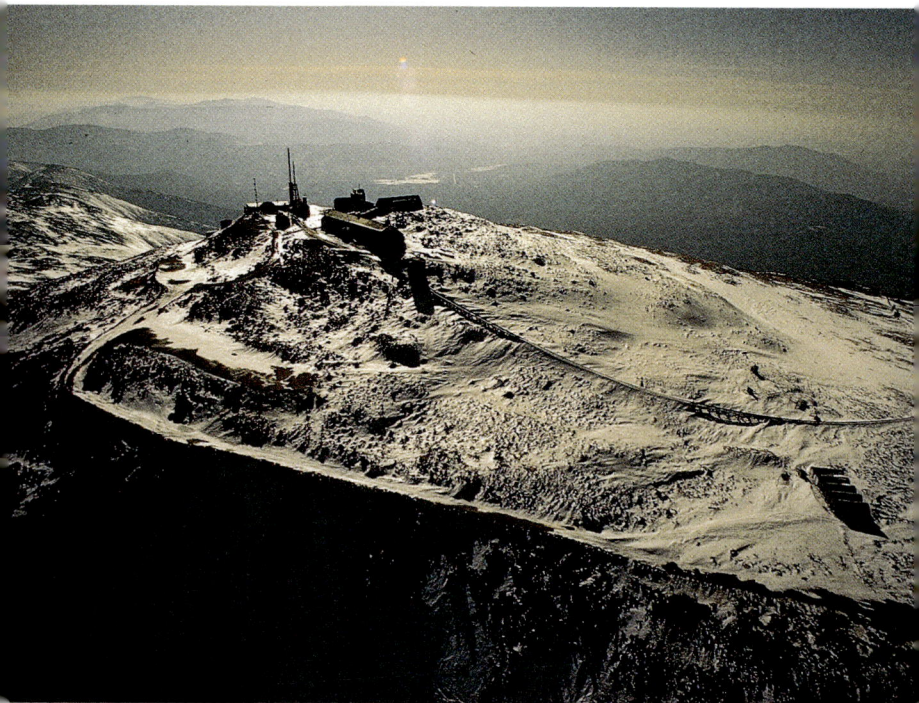

At the top of Mount Washington are a number of buildings and attractions. So even in bad weather—nearly always the case—a trip to the "City Among the Clouds" can be fun.

Avalanche!

9   Another danger on Mount Washington is falling snow. Snow piles up in the several great ravines[5] of this broad-shouldered mountain. The most famous ravine is Tuckerman Ravine, known for its excellent skiing conditions.

10   Once in a while, there is an avalanche. Anyone caught in this falling snow may be buried alive. In 1996, two skiers were killed by an avalanche in a ravine just south of Tuckerman. Even the ravine's name—the Gulf of Slides—seems a warning of sorts.

A Great Mountain

11   Although visitors must be careful when they hike Mount Washington, it is still a great mountain. On a clear day—which is rare—a person can see 100 miles from the top.

12   The first person to climb Mount Washington was Darby Field, who scaled the peak in 1642. In 1784, the mountain was named in honor of U.S. President George Washington. Of the area's mountains, known as the Presidential Range, Mount Washington is the highest. Nearby mountains in this range are also named after U.S. presidents: Adams, Madison, Lincoln, and so on.

---

[5] ravine: a deep, narrow crack or passage in the earth's surface

Although Mount Clinton is not too far from these peaks, it wasn't named for President Bill Clinton.

Getting to the Top

13 Despite its fierce weather, Mount Washington draws thousands of tourists each year. Many hike, but some drive up the paved toll road to the top. Plenty of parking awaits visitors once they get there.

14 The 3-mile-long Cog Railway, built in 1869, also brings tourists to the top of the mountain. This railway was viewed as one of the great marvels[6] of the 19th century. At times, the little train seems to be going straight up. No other train in the United States has a steeper slope.

15 No matter how people get to the mountaintop, they find plenty of company when they arrive. This can be a bit of a shock to hikers. They spend three or four hours climbing through the woods and over rocks to reach the top. But they don't find peace and quiet there. To their surprise, they meet the hundreds of tourists who drove up in their cars.

16 The summit[7] of Mount Washington can make a tourist feel right at home. It has restrooms, food service, gift shops, a post office, and a museum. Other features are a major weather and research

---

[6] marvel: something that causes great wonder
[7] summit: the top or highest point

station, a lookout center, and even a TV tower. These buildings, activities, and conveniences may be why the top of Mount Washington is sometimes called the "City Among the Clouds."

17   Visitors might reach the top of Mount Washington on foot, by car, or by rail. The temperature there might be 60 degrees above zero or 20 degrees below. The view might be 100 miles or 100 feet, the day clear or thick with fog. Because of these extremes, Mount Washington is full of surprises. It's no wonder that the top of the region's highest peak will seem like a different place with each visit!

QUESTIONS

1. Why is it said that Mount Washington has the worst weather in the world?
2. What makes this fairly small mountain so deadly?
3. What is hypothermia?
4. Name three ways people can reach the top of Mount Washington.
5. Why is Mount Washington's peak sometimes called the "City among the Clouds"?

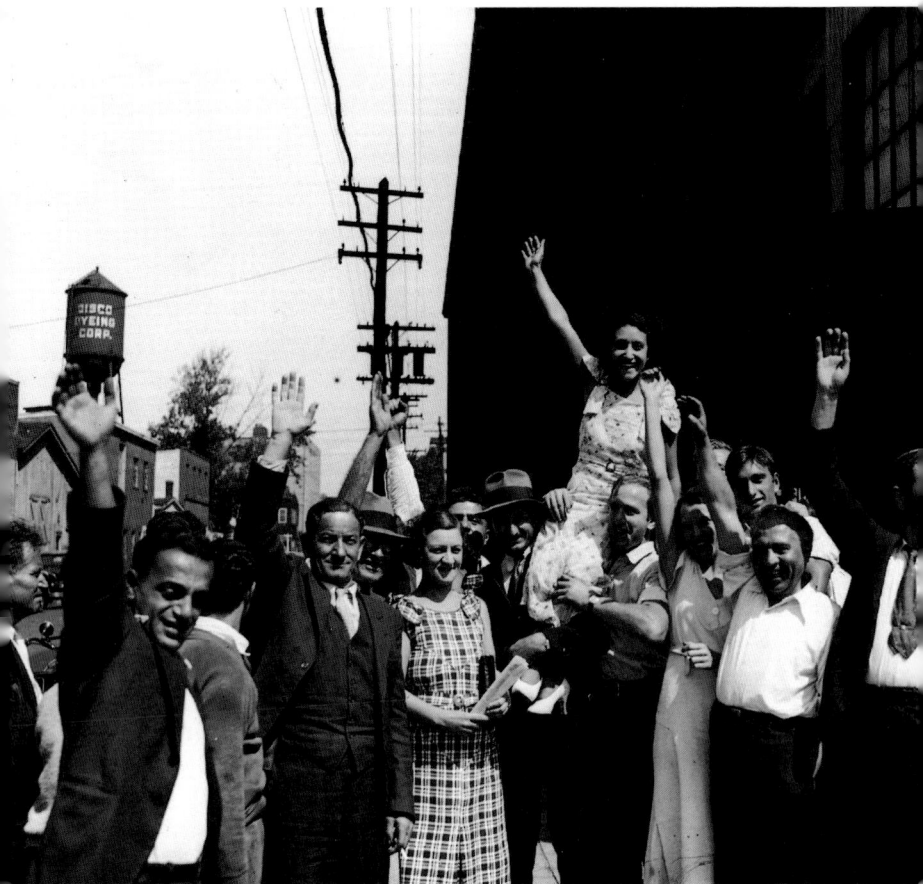

In this 1934 photo, workers in a New Jersey silk factory go on strike for better wages.

FIGHTING FOR
Minimum Wage

Why have people always disagreed about the minimum wage law?

1   In 1938, Congress passed the Fair Labor Standards[1] Act. Part of this law included setting a minimum wage. The wage was set at 25 cents an hour. Of course, 25 cents had much more buying power in 1938 than it does today.

2   The new law didn't cover all United States workers—only about one worker in five. Still, the law made some employers pay their workers at least 25 cents an hour. Many business owners were unhappy about having to obey the law.

Argument Against a Minimum Wage

3   How are wage rates set? In the United States, they are set by the free market. In other words,

---

[1] standard: a measure that something has to reach to be satisfactory

a worker is "free" to sell his or her labor. An employer is "free" to buy that labor. Both employer and worker must agree on its price or wage. This kind of freedom is at the heart of the free market system. No one *has* to buy or sell services if he or she doesn't want to.

4 From the start, many employers fought the minimum wage law. They thought that the amount they paid their workers was none of the government's business. For these employers, the issue was freedom.

5 At first, the U.S. Supreme Court agreed. By 1923, 15 states had their own minimum wage laws, but the Supreme Court then struck them all down. The reason was simple: state governments could not restrict[2] the free-market system.

The Great Depression[3]

6 The Great Depression was a tough time. One third of all workers could not find jobs. Many of those who had jobs were poorly paid. They worked in "sweatshops," so named because of their low pay, long hours, and unsafe working conditions. The workers, often women and children, were paid only 10 or 15 cents an hour.

---

[2] restrict: limit or keep inside a boundary
[3] Great Depression: the period of very low business activity and loss of money worldwide brought on by the United States stock market crash of 1929

7   That amount of money was not enough to live on. Workers began to ask the government to do something. For them, setting a minimum wage was not a question of freedom but one of justice. It seemed unfair to pay people so little. By 1938, these workers had won the argument. The Fair Labor Standards Act was passed. This time the Supreme Court let it stand.

New Arguments

8   The minimum wage is set at a higher rate than a rate the free market would set. It has to be that way; if the rate weren't higher, the minimum wage would serve no purpose. There would be no need for such a law.

9   However, setting the minimum wage rate higher than the free-market rate leads to a new argument against having the law: it costs jobs. This job loss happens

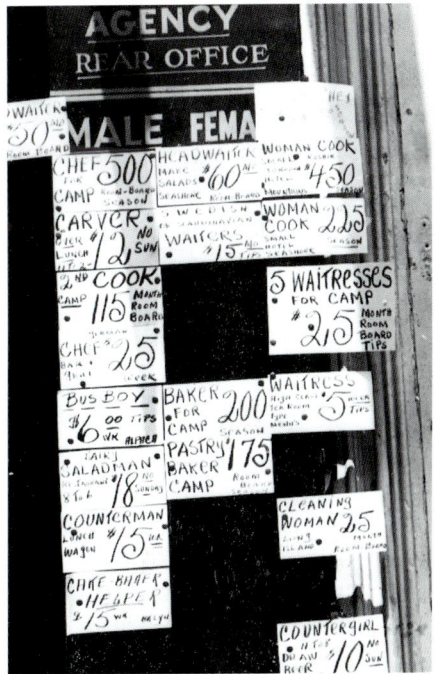

This employment agency's job ads show the low wage scales common in the 1930s, the time of the Great Depression.

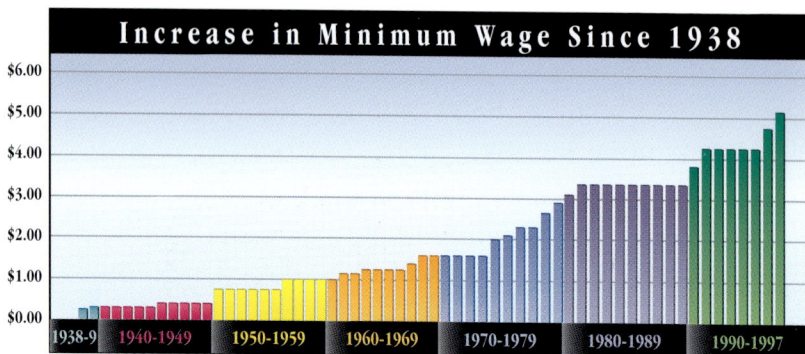

Increase in Minimum Wage Since 1938

The minimum wage has risen over the years. Although the original fight for a minimum wage was won in 1938, pay rates and types of work covered by law are still points of debate.

because some employers cannot afford to pay the higher, or minimum, wage. For example, an employer might have workers on jobs that pay the lower, or free-market, rate. But the employer can't afford to pay that same number of workers a higher wage—the minimum wage fixed by law. To obey the law, the employer must then reduce the number of jobs (and the workers who hold them) to what the company can support.

Since 1938

10　The minimum wage is, of course, no longer 25 cents an hour. Over the years it has been raised slowly to keep up with the rising cost of living.[4] In 1950, Congress increased the rate to 75 cents an hour. By 1968, it was $1.60 an hour. And by 1991, it was $4.25 an hour.

---

[4] cost of living: the usual cost of basic things people need, such as food, clothing, and a place to live

11   A new minimum wage law passed in 1996 that called for a two-step raise. The minimum wage first went up to $4.75 an hour. Then, in 1997, it rose to $5.15 an hour. The 1996 law boosted the wages of about 10 million workers.

12   But what about all of those lost jobs? One argument against the recent increases was that they would hurt the job outlook for teenaged workers. Not many employers want to pay $5.15 an hour to unskilled workers, many of whom are teens. The new law tried to answer that complaint by setting a lower wage for workers under age 20. These teens could earn $4.25 an hour for 90 days. After 90 days, the teenage workers would get the standard[5] minimum wage of $5.15 an hour.

13   Another major change since 1938 is that far more types of work pay the minimum wage than ever before. Certain farmworkers, for example, are now covered under the minimum wage law for the first time. So are some workers in hotels, retail [rē′tāl] stores, and restaurants.

Support of Minimum Wage

14   In politics, raising the minimum wage rate is often a popular thing to do. Democrats have voted for such raises, and so have many Republicans. Since President Franklin Roosevelt,

---

[5] standard: normal

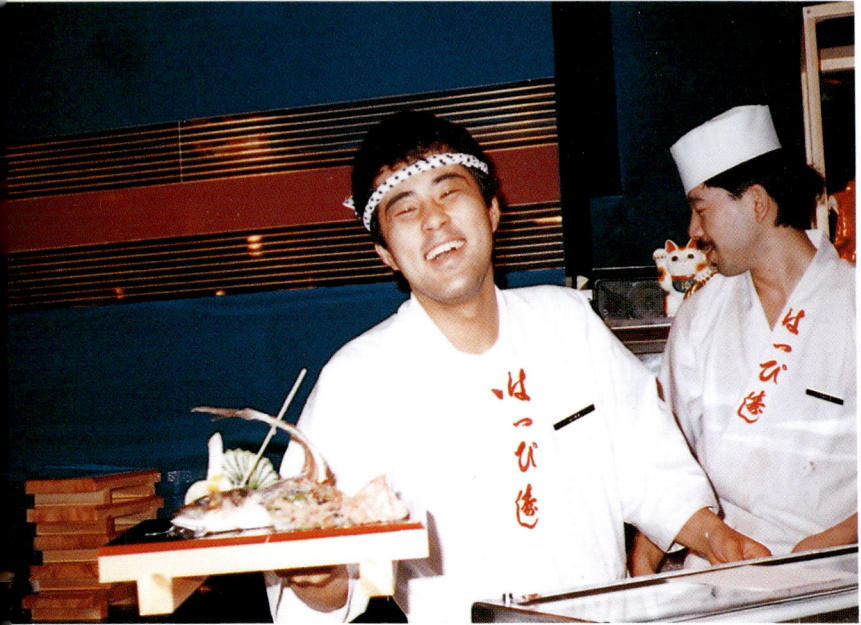

Changes to the minimum wage law covered more and more types of workers, like this restaurant server, for the first time.

a Democrat, signed the first minimum wage law (in 1938), eight U.S. presidents have signed wage hike bills into law. The three Republicans on that list are Dwight Eisenhower, Richard Nixon, and George Bush.

15   The minimum wage law remains controversial[6] [kŏn trə vûr′shəl]. But the fight is no longer about the law itself. That war has been won. The fight these days is about the actual wage rate, which will always be a subject for debate.

---

[6] controversial: something that causes people to disagree and take different sides

QUESTIONS

1. What is the Fair Labor Standards Act?
2. Why did some people at first fight against the minimum wage?
3. What idea turned the Supreme Court in favor of the minimum wage law?
4. How has the minimum wage law changed since 1938?
5. Why will people keep arguing about the minimum wage law?

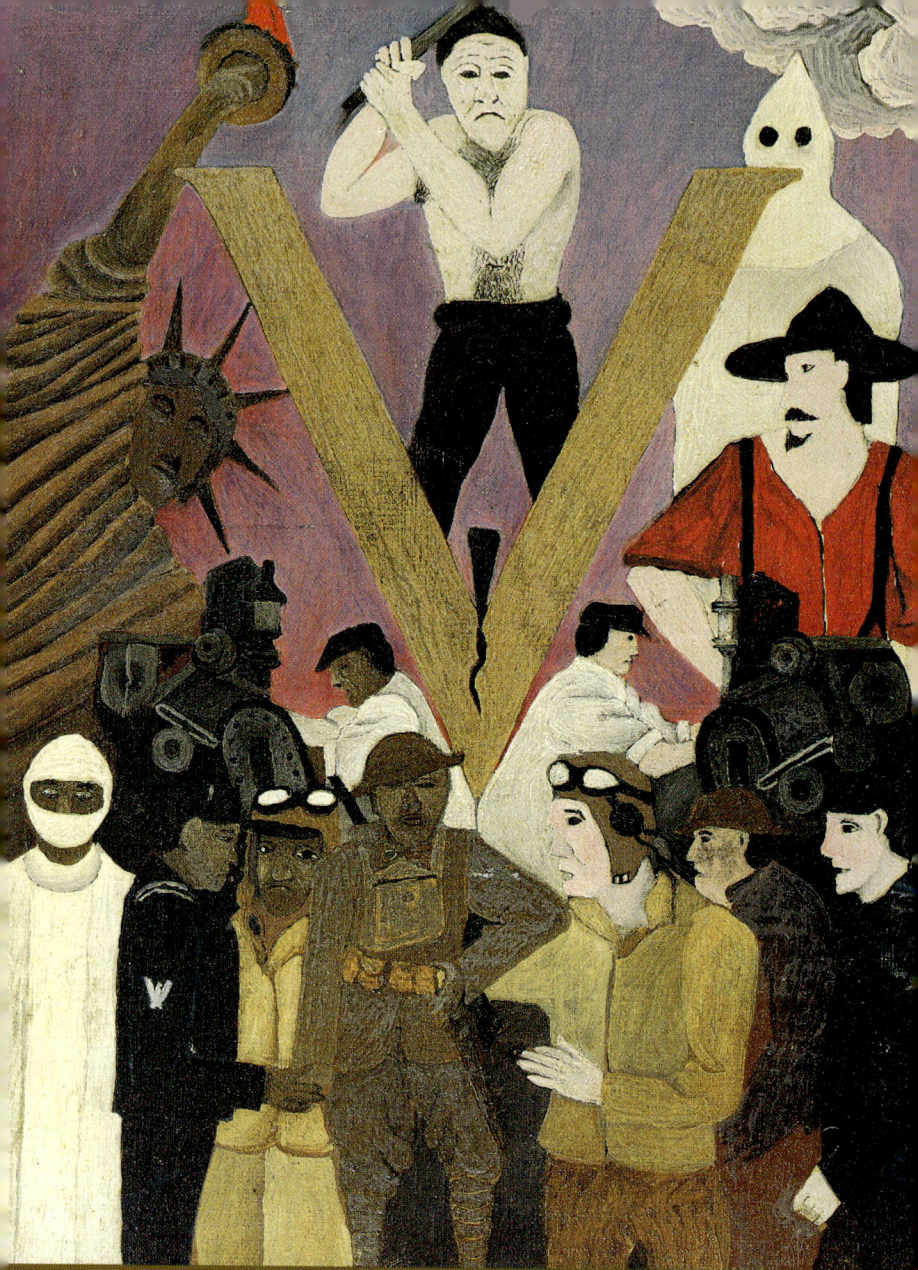

Mr. Prejudice (1943) reflects the important life events that shaped the outlook of African-American artist Horace Pippin.

Works from the Heart

Who was Horace Pippin?
What is special about his art?

1   In the spring of 1937, two men were walking through West Chester, Pennsylvania. One man was N.C. Wyeth, a famous artist. The other was Christian Brinton, an expert art critic. The men spotted a painting in the window of a shoe repair shop. They could tell that the artist had not had painting lessons. But there was something special about the painting.

2   Brinton went to visit the artist, who lived nearby. The artist was Horace Pippin, and he was 49 years old. Pippin had taught himself to paint. And painting had changed his life.

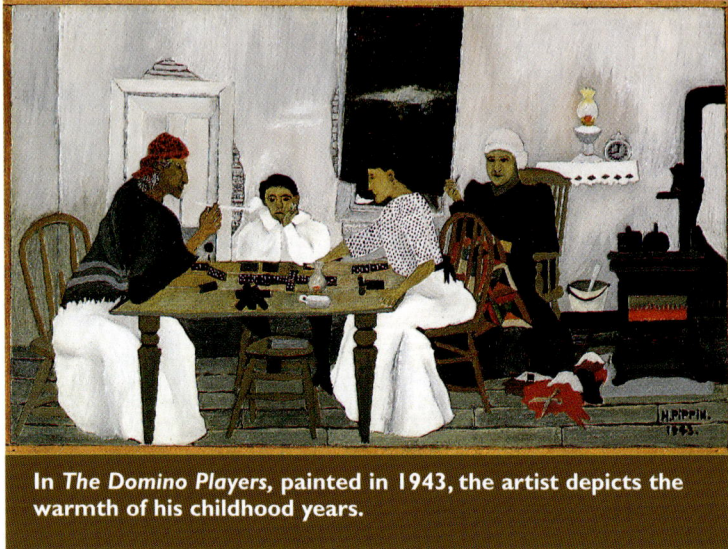

In *The Domino Players,* painted in 1943, the artist depicts the warmth of his childhood years.

Pippin's Early Life

3   Pippin was born in West Chester in 1888. His grandparents had been slaves, and his parents were household workers. The family moved to Goshen, New York, when Pippin was three.

4   Pippin showed a talent for art even as a child. On spelling tests, he drew pictures of the words. At age 10, Pippin entered a picture in a magazine contest and won a prize.

5   Pippin dropped out of school at age 14. He went to work in a coal yard, then at a feed store. For seven years, he worked as a hotel porter. In 1912, Pippin moved to New Jersey, where he worked as a furniture packer and an iron molder.

A World War I Soldier

6   When Horace Pippin was 29, his life changed forever. That year, the United States entered World War I. American troops fought the Germans in Europe. Pippin joined the army and was sent to France. His regiment, the 369th Infantry, was an all-black unit known for its courage. The Germans called these soldiers the "Hell Fighters." The 369th fought in the trenches[1] on the front lines for many months.

7   Life in the trenches was terrible. Constant rain soaked the soldiers to the skin. Pippin wrote that sometimes he was unable to take off his shoes for 20 days at a time. Bombshells burst overhead night and day. And there was the ever-present danger of a German poison-gas attack.

8   Pippin wrote of his experiences in notebooks. The notebooks clearly show the horrors of war. In them, Pippin also drew pictures to illustrate his stories. They show soldiers wearing gas masks during an attack. They show bombshells exploding in the air and dogfights[2] between fighter planes.

9   On a mission, 3 of the 10 men in Pippin's squad were killed in hand-to-hand combat. But

---

[1] trench: a long ditch dug by soldiers for protection and for a base from which to attack the enemy

[2] dogfight: a gunfight between two fighter planes flying at close range

the squad came out on top. They killed 9 of the 10 German soldiers who were attacking.

10   One day, Pippin was shot in the neck, shoulder, and right arm. He fell into a deep shell hole.[3] He was trapped by gunfire and lost a lot of blood. A soldier came to help, but he was shot too and fell on top of Pippin. Pippin could not move. After many hours in heavy rain, Pippin was rescued. But he lay on a stretcher overnight in the pouring rain. The next day, he was finally taken to a hospital.

11   His wounds left Pippin physically shattered. He had to have a steel plate put in his shoulder. His right arm was paralyzed[4] [păr′ ə līzd].

12   The war left Pippin mentally shattered as well. For the rest of his life, he was haunted by memories of life and death in the trenches.

After the War

13   In 1920, Pippin married Jennie Giles, a widow with a young son. They made their home in a small brick house in West Chester. She took in laundry. He did light work and got a small disability pension.[5]

---

[3] shell hole: a crater in the ground caused by an exploding bombshell

[4] paralyzed: not able to move

[5] disability pension: a fixed amount of money granted by the government to soldiers wounded in a war

14   Pippin was a tall, strong man with many interests. He liked people and had a good sense of humor. After the war, however, he often became depressed. As therapy for his arm, and to keep his spirits up, Pippin returned to art.

15   His first experiments were with charcoal drawings on cigar boxes. He did not like the outcome. Next, Pippin used a hot poker to burn pictures into wood. He held the poker in his right hand.

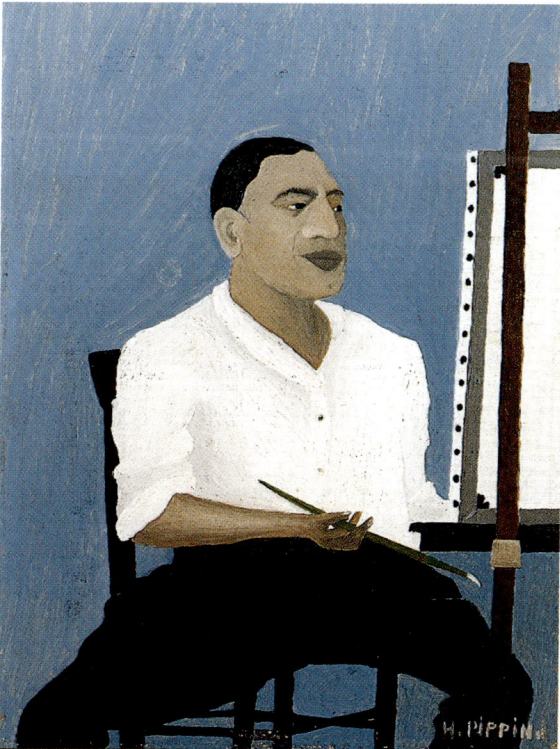

Pippin, here in a self-portrait from 1941, returned to painting to strengthen his right arm, wounded in war.

Because his right arm was weak, Pippin braced the hand on his knee. With his left hand, he moved the wood against the poker's hot tip. Pippin used this method for more than 12 years. "It brought me back to my old self," he said.

16   By the late 1920s, Pippin's right arm was stronger. He took up oil painting, working in a small room under an unshaded light bulb. He used cheap, handy materials such as house paint.

17   Oil painting was a slow, painful process for Pippin. He held the brush in his right hand and guided it across the canvas with his left hand. He painted layer over layer until he liked what he saw. It took him three years—and at least 100 coats of paint—to complete his first oil painting.

18   Pippin once said, "The war brought out all the art in me. I came home with all of it in my mind, and I paint from it today." His first painting, completed in 1930, is called *The End of the War: Starting Home*. It shows German soldiers surrendering to black American troops. It is not a celebration of victory. Rather, it is a statement about the cruelty of war.

Success

19   Pippin kept painting about his war experiences. Sometimes he traded his art for goods from stores. Other times he put art up for sale in store windows. Few people took the paintings seriously.

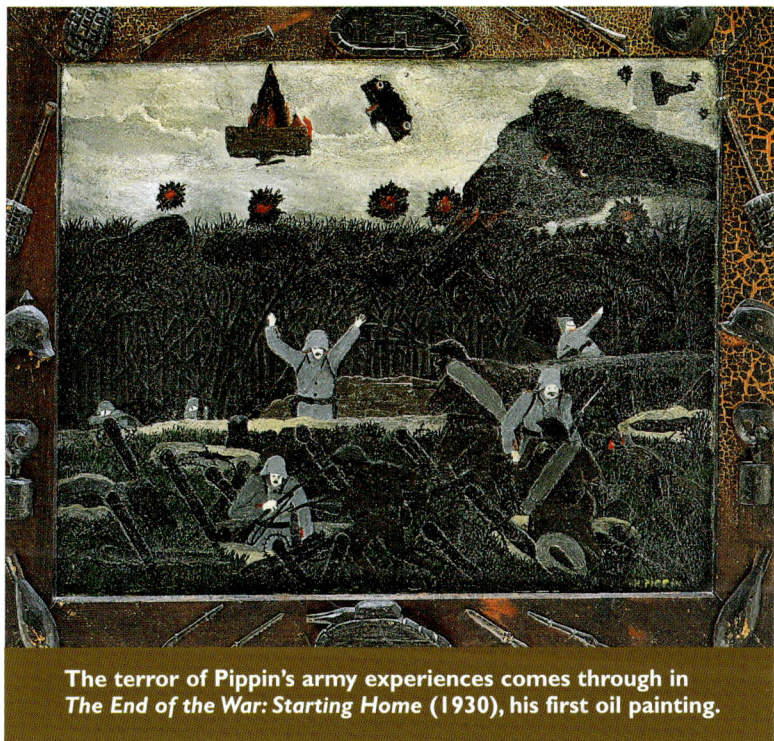

The terror of Pippin's army experiences comes through in *The End of the War: Starting Home* (1930), his first oil painting.

20   In 1935, Pippin began to paint other subjects. *Cabin in the Cotton I* shows a rustic home in a field of cotton. This is the painting that Wyeth and Brinton saw in the shoeshop window.

21   Brinton worked hard to spread the word about Pippin's paintings. In 1938, he arranged for some of Pippin's work to appear in a museum show. The show, called "Masters of Modern Popular Painting," began at the Museum of Modern Art in New York City. Then it moved to museums across the country. Pippin was on his way to success.

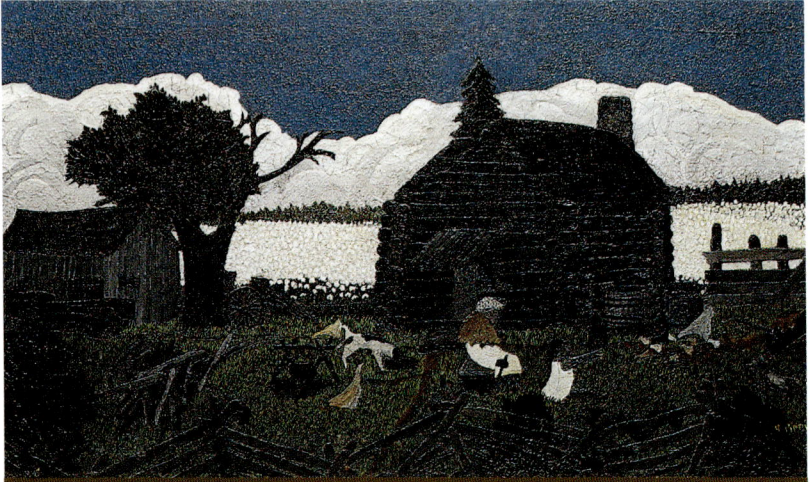

Cabin in the Cotton I, from 1935, shows a simple country house against a sea of cotton. It is the painting that opened the doors of the art world to Pippin.

22   Pippin's career got a big boost when Robert Carlen of Philadelphia became his dealer. Carlen gave Pippin good materials to work with. He also told other museums and private collectors about Pippin's work.

23   In 1940, Carlen arranged Pippin's first one-man show. The show got very good reviews, and the paintings sold quickly. Theater and movie stars became fans of Pippin's work. Museums across the country bought his paintings.

24   Pippin became known as an important artist in the "folk art" movement. He painted portraits of people and scenes from everyday life. He also painted landscapes and common items such as fruit or flowers.

Following His Heart

25 Describing his art, Pippin said that his paintings were like photographs. He painted each subject "exactly the way it is and exactly the way I see it." He painted mainly from memory and imagination. "Pictures just come to my mind," he once said, "and then I tell my heart to go ahead."

26   Sadly, Horace Pippin could not enjoy his fame for long. He died in 1946, just nine years after being discovered. Today, Pippin remains a popular and respected folk artist. He is also an inspiration. He was an artist with no formal art training. He was a man who painted to heal his paralyzed arm. He was a man who followed his heart. ◈

QUESTIONS

1. Who was Horace Pippin?
2. What happened to Pippin during World War I?
3. Why did Pippin return to art after the war?
4. How was Pippin discovered by the art world?
5. In what way are Pippin's paintings like photographs?

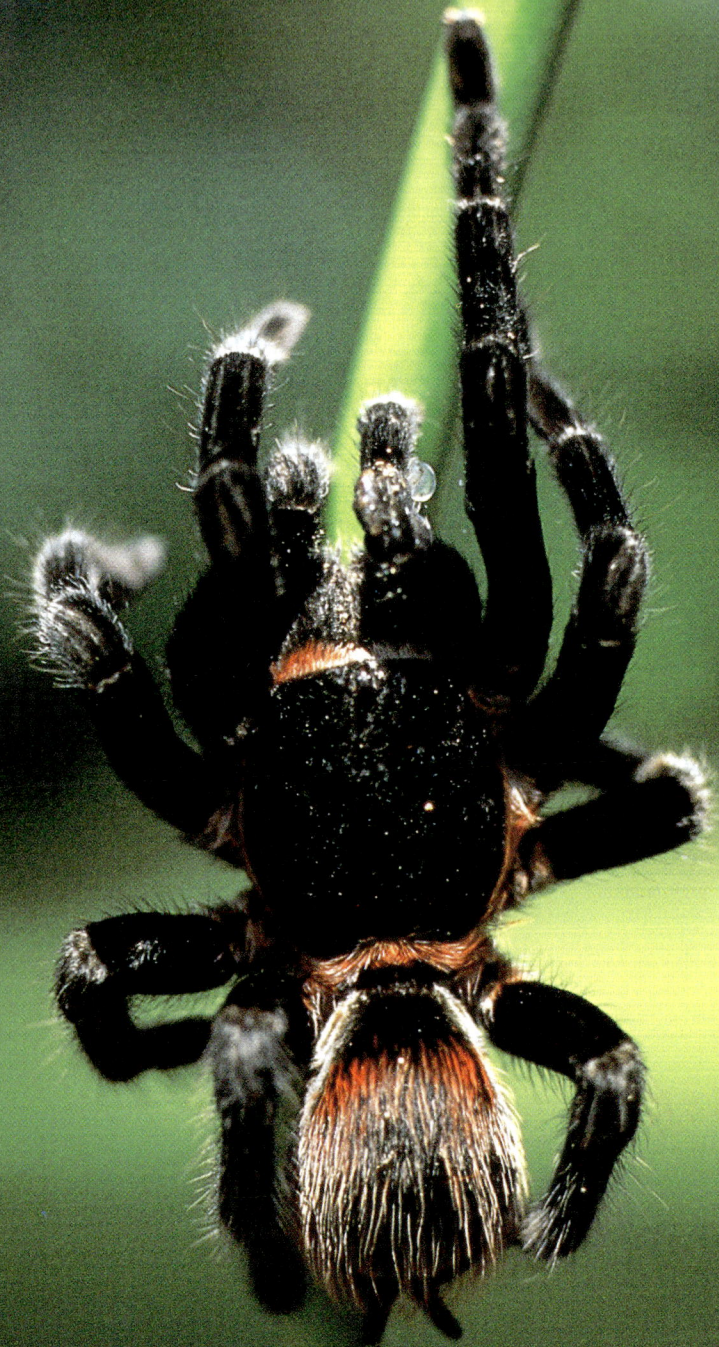

A TARANTULA
Big Hairy Deal

Are tarantulas really as dangerous as they look?

1   Tarantulas [tə răn′chə ləz] are the largest spiders on Earth. Some of them grow to be the size of a person's hand. A few get even bigger than that. The largest ones can be the size of a dinner plate.

2   Maybe it's their size that makes tarantulas so scary. Or maybe it's their hairy bodies. Their eight beady eyes do nothing to calm the nerves, either. Then there are those two large fangs[1] filled with venom[2] [věn′əm]. All in all, tarantulas look quite fearsome, so they have been portrayed as aggressive killers. In movies and on TV, tarantulas have long been a symbol of death. Certain folklore may also play a part in the "bad rap" these creatures have had to live with through the ages.

---

[1] fang: a long, sharp tooth used in biting or poisoning
[2] venom: poison from an animal such as a spider or snake

While not exactly cuddly, tarantulas are not really monsters whose bite spells certain death, either.

3   The word *tarantula* comes from a large spider
found near Taranto, a city in southern Italy.
People once thought that a bite from this spider
caused a sickness called *tarantism* [tăr′ ən tĭz əm].
People with this illness were said to leap into
the air and run wildly, making odd noises. The
best cure in that day was a lively folk dance.
The dance became known as the *tarantella,* which
is still performed today—but not to cure disease!

Interesting but not Deadly

4   The truth about tarantulas is less frightening
than the myths of old would have you think.
Tarantulas *do* kill with their venom, but they don't

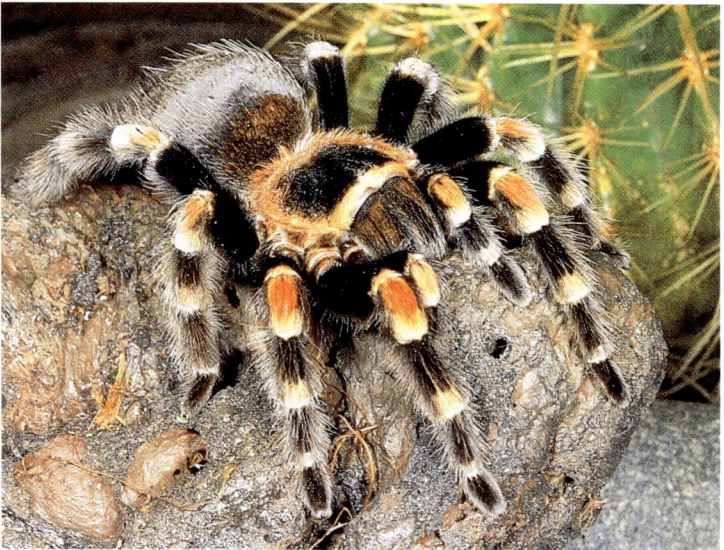

**A tarantula relies on all that hair and a loud hissing sound
for self-defense. The poor devil is as often the hunted as
the hunter.**

kill humans. Their venom is designed mostly for beetles and grasshoppers. It can't disable anything larger than a mouse or bat. Tarantulas rarely bite humans. When they do, the bite is no worse than a wasp sting.

5   Although tarantulas do not hunt humans, they are still fascinating. Scientists have found about 800 kinds, which live mostly in warm climates. They live in the American Southwest, Europe, and Asia. In fact, they live on every continent but Antarctica. Many tarantulas make their homes in rain forests. Scientists think that these forests hold many unknown species of tarantulas.

As Blind as a . . . Tarantula?

6   All tarantulas share certain features. They have long, hairy legs and thick, hairy bodies. Despite their many eyes, tarantulas do not see well. In this case, more is not better. Tarantulas must rely on other senses to help them get what they need.

7   Most important of these is the spiders' sense of touch. Tarantulas travel by feeling their way along. They find prey by picking up vibrations made by the prey as it moves. All the hairs on the tarantulas' bodies help them sense these vibrations. The hairs move with even the slightest breeze. So when their hairs start vibrating, tarantulas know the air is swirling. That motion usually signals something nearby: dinner is on the way.

8   Tarantulas use one other trick as well. They
spin silk threads near their burrows. If a creature
hits one of these threads, the thread jiggles. The
jiggling alerts the tarantula that food is nearby.

A Liquid Diet

9   A tarantula hunts for food at night. Once it finds
its prey, the spider moves fast. It sinks its fangs
deep into the victim's body, paralyzing it with
venom. Then the tarantula can take its time. It
often drags its prey back to its burrow or to some
other safe place. Then it does something odd.
Since a tarantula cannot eat solid food, it pumps
digestive[3] [dĭ jĕs′ tĭv] fluids onto its victim. These
fluids, which look like many wet threads of silk,
come from silk glands at the rear of the spider.
The silken juices cover the victim and wrap
around it. Soon the flesh of the victim
dissolves[4] into liquid. The spider then sucks out
the liquids from the victim. Feeding can go on
for hours, until nothing is left of the victim but
a dry husk.[5]

10   In the winter, tarantulas hibernate.[6] In the
summer, they eat only about once a week. If they

---

[3] digestive: relating to the process of converting food to
simpler forms for use by the body
[4] dissolve: to melt down to a liquid
[5] husk: a thin, dry, outer covering or shell
[6] hibernate: to spend the winter sleeping or resting

must, they can go much longer than that without a meal. One large female was kept away from food for a long time. After two years, she was still alive.

The Hunter is Hunted

11 Tarantulas eat many small creatures but may themselves be eaten by other animals. Their worst enemy is the female Pepsis [pĕp′sĭs] wasp. The Pepsis is a big wasp—the largest in the world. Because of its size and diet, it is nicknamed the "tarantula hawk."

A tarantula's venom comes from little bulbs inside the spider's hollow fangs. The fangs stick out of two large jaws below the eyes.

12 Although large for a wasp, the Pepsis is still smaller than a tarantula. Sometimes it is much, much smaller. A tarantula may weigh ten times as much as a Pepsis, but that doesn't stop a fighting wasp. She will swoop down and try to sting a tarantula at the base of a leg. The tarantula, meanwhile, tries to bite the wasp. The battle can be fierce, and the stakes are high. The loser, after all, ends up dead.

13 If the wasp wins, she lays a single egg on top of the dead tarantula. Then she buries the spider. When the egg hatches, the baby wasp finds itself sitting on its first meal!

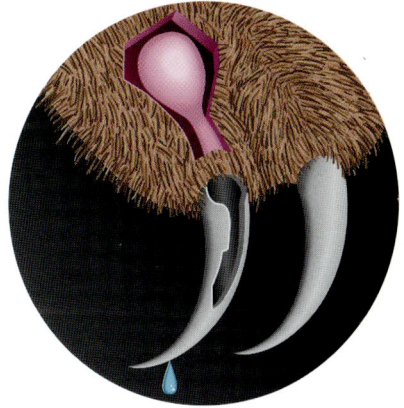

Self-Defense

14 Tarantulas have several ways to protect themselves from wasps and other enemies. One defense they use is a loud hissing sound to scare enemies away. Tarantulas make the hissing noise by rubbing their legs together. The spider's leg hairs produce the sound.

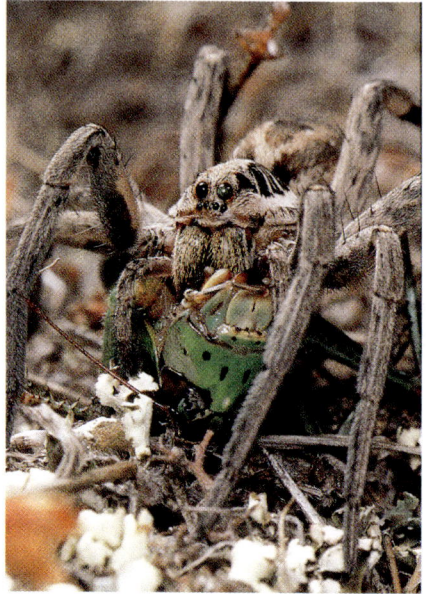

A tarantula feasts on a dinner of fresh beetle. Notice that the spider has sunk its fangs inside the victim.

15 Hair also plays a role in a second defense. When threatened, tarantulas rub their back legs over their bellies, rubbing off many hairs. These hairs fly through the air, and some may hit the enemy. They cause a strong burning or itching feeling on the enemy's skin. Mice that inhale these hairs have died from their effects.

16 A tarantula has a third and final defense. As a last resort, it will use its huge fangs to bite an attacker that tries to get away.

Popular Pets

17 Some people say that the more they learn about tarantulas, the more they like them. That may be why tarantulas are popular in pet stores. More and more people are buying them. Owners praise tarantulas as wonderful pets. Tarantulas don't bark like dogs, eat a lot, smell, make messes, or take up much room. But they are quite interesting to watch.

18 Even so, it is hard to shake the old image of tarantulas as symbols of terror. Their place on the Halloween scene ranks with the likes of vampires and rattling skeletons. So if the thought of a tarantula on the loose makes you cringe,[7] you're not alone. Just remember that a tarantula's "bark" is far worse than its bite!

QUESTIONS

1. How did tarantulas get their name?
2. Where do tarantulas live?
3. How does a tarantula find food?
4. How does a Pepsis wasp act toward a tarantula?
5. Name three ways a tarantula can defend itself from enemies?

---

[7] cringe: to shrink in fear

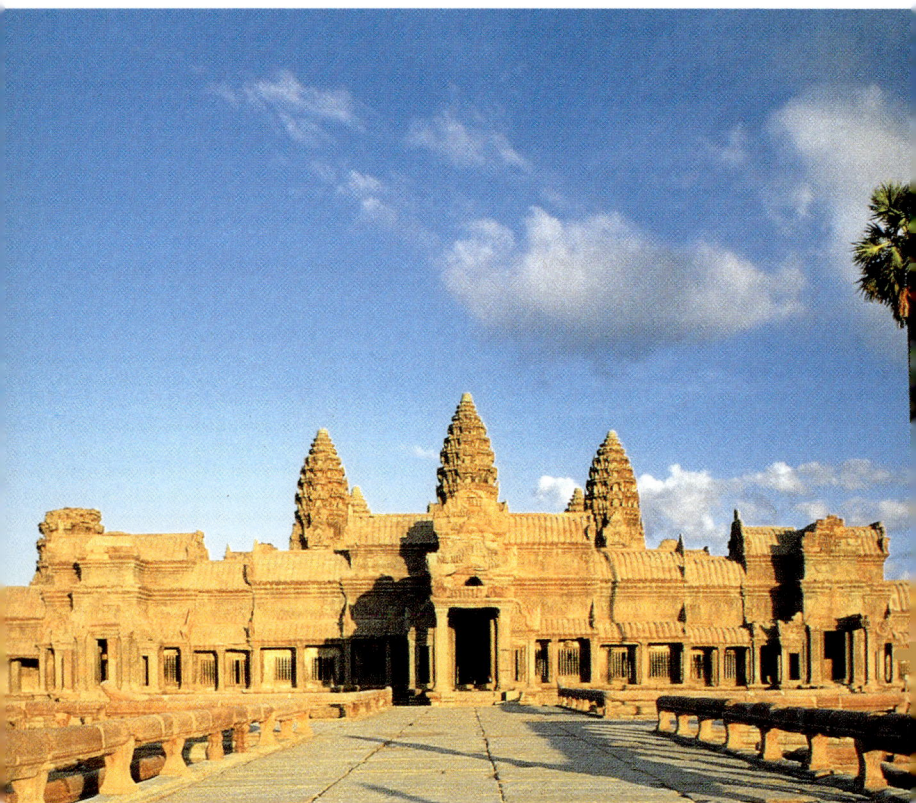

Built as a Hindu Temple, Angkor Wat is the largest religious monument in the world.

CAMBODIA'S
GRAND TEMPLE

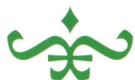

*What makes Angkor Wat
one of the world's great treasures?*

1 Angkor Wat [ăng′kōr wăt] is among the most important structures in the world. It is in the same class as the Great Wall of China and the pyramids of Egypt. Yet until recently, it was unknown to most people. Little by little, the world is starting to see what a treasure Angkor Wat really is.

Building the Temple

2 The people of Cambodia are known as Khmer [kə mâr′]. In the ninth century, they decided to build a new capital and chose a place in north-western Cambodia. The Khmer called their city *Angkor,* which means "capital." The city was built around a temple on a hill. At that time in history, the Khmer practiced the Hindu religion. They believed that a temple was the center of the world.

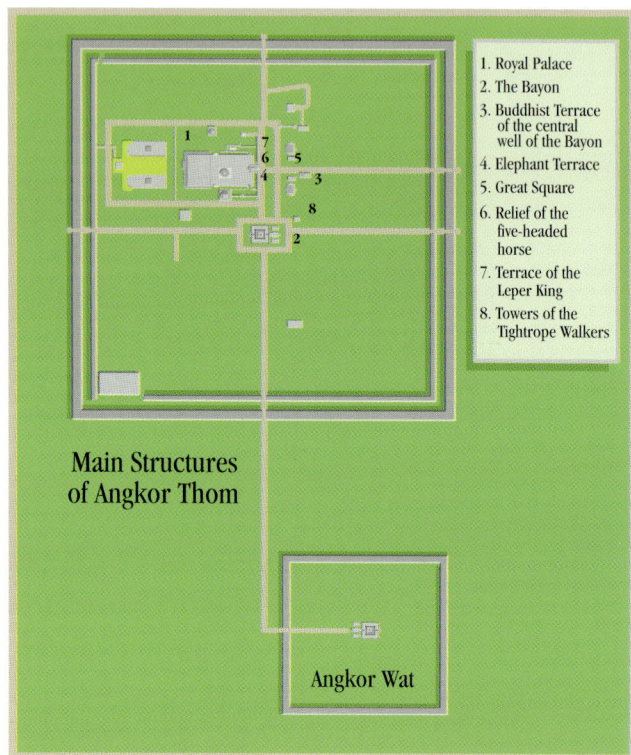

1. Royal Palace
2. The Bayon
3. Buddhist Terrace of the central well of the Bayon
4. Elephant Terrace
5. Great Square
6. Relief of the five-headed horse
7. Terrace of the Leper King
8. Towers of the Tightrope Walkers

Main Structures of Angkor Thom

Angkor Wat

The plan above shows the location of Angkor Wat and the main palaces and temples of the ancient Khmer capital. Even the interesting names of these structures hint at the rich cultural and religious history of Cambodia.

3   Over the years, Khmer kings added many more temples, forming a large group of buildings. These buildings extended 15 miles from east to west and 8 miles from north to south. The most magnificent building was Angkor Wat. (The word *wat* means "temple.") Angkor Wat was built by King Suryavarman II, who ruled in the early twelfth century.

4   Angkor Wat is the largest temple in the world. Built of stone, the stunning structure stands 200 feet high. A moat[1] 2 1/2-miles wide surrounds the temple.

5   Everything about the temple's design was inspired by Hindu beliefs. For example, the temple's five lotus[2]-shaped towers stand for mountains. Hindus believe that mountains are the dwelling places of the gods. The large moat around the temple is a symbol for the oceans of the world. Beyond these "oceans" lies the outside world. The moat removes and protects the temple from the rest of the world—a design meant to honor the gods. To reach the temple requires crossing a 617-foot bridge. The temple walls are covered with fine sculptures, which show scenes from Hindu stories.

Neglect and Decay

6   In 1177, Angkor was attacked. A neighboring group of people sacked[3] the city. The event made King Jayavarman VII, who ruled at that time, believe that the Hindu gods had failed him.

---

[1] moat: a ditch filled with water that surrounds a castle or old, important structure

[2] lotus: a plant from southern Asia that grows in water and has big leaves and pink flowers.

[3] sacked: stole goods of a captured city or town

So he built a new capital nearby called Angkor Thom [tŏm] and dedicated it to Buddhism [bo͞o ′dĭz əm]. Angkor Wat then became a Buddhist shrine, and Buddhist art replaced some of its Hindu art.

7   In spite of the King's efforts, the Khmer empire became weak anyway. Armies from Thailand [tī′lănd] kept attacking Angkor. At last, in 1431, these enemy armies captured the city of Angkor. The Khmer abandoned the city and moved south for safety. Certain monks continued to use Angkor Wat for a while. Later, the surrounding jungle slowly overgrew the city and its many temples. Left to the forces of nature, Angkor began to decay. Its temples fell to ruins.

8   That was how things stayed for more than 400 years. Then, in 1860, a French explorer "discovered" the city, and French scholars began to research the temples' history. The findings soon led others to understand that the temples were worth saving. By the early 1900s, a large-scale program to restore the temples had begun.

9   World Wars I and II slowed work on the temples. Later, the war in Vietnam spilled into Cambodia. Bombs and other ground fighting destroyed much of the country. In spite of all the trouble, Angkor Wat suffered only a few bullet holes. The real damage to it had happened through neglect.

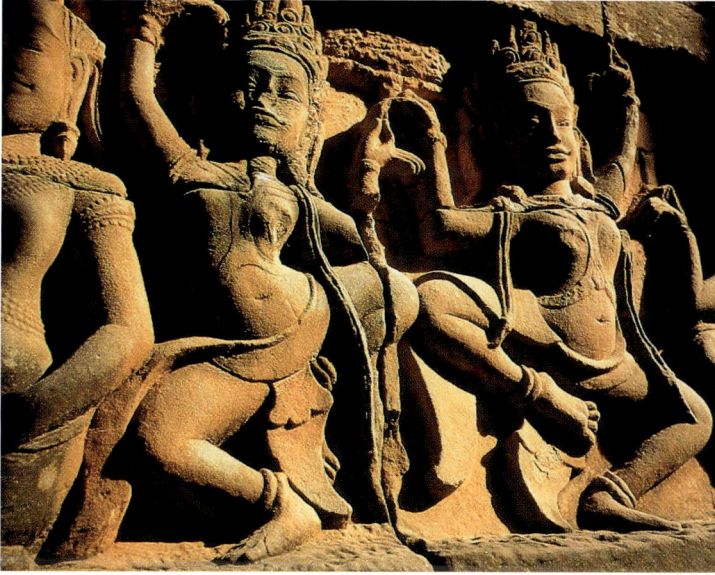

Among the group of buildings in the Angkor Wat area is the Terrace of the Leper King. The sculptures show scenes from Hindu legend.

Angkor Wat Today

10   Most of Angkor Wat has been saved. It took much work and a great amount of concrete. The many years of neglect had damaged the temple's foundation. A new concrete foundation had to be poured under the buildings. To support the old sandstone blocks, it was necessary to also build new inside walls of concrete.

11   The years of chaos[4] [kā′ŏs] and war caused another form of damage—theft. It happened often during the late 1970s, when Pol Pot [pŏl pŏt′] ruled Cambodia. During Pol Pot's

---

[4] chaos: total disorder or confusion

reign of terror, Cambodian communists—called the Khmer Rouge [kə mâr′ rōōzh]—killed more than 1 million Cambodians. Pol Pot's soldiers also tore through Angkor Wat, taking more than 3,500 priceless works of art. They sold most of these pieces to private dealers in Bangkok.

12   For all it has been through, Angkor Wat remains a treasure. Rising grandly out of the jungle, the temple is an important link to Cambodia's past. It also shows the beauty and great depth of the Hindu religion.

A New Problem

13   The importance of Angkor Wat, however, has caused a major dilemma[5] in recent years. Should the temple be protected as a holy shrine, or should it be further opened to tourists?

14   It is not an easy choice. Cambodia is a very poor country; its people could use the money that the tourist trade would bring in. In 1986, Angkor Wat drew only 565 tourists. Ten years later, in 1996, more than 70,000 visitors flocked to see the temple. Such interest meant a large increase in tourist dollars. Now developers want to pave the way for even more tourists in the years to come. They have planned to build luxury hotels along the road leading to Angkor.

---

[5] dilemma: a problem that requires a choice between two equal courses of action

These builders also put pressure on Cambodian officials to relax laws that limit the areas for building.

15   Not all Cambodians like the changes that are taking place. Tourists have started to leave their mark on Angkor Wat already. Trash litters the grounds. Even worse, some tourists have written graffiti on the temple walls.

16   Many Cambodians are speaking out against the tourist trade. They don't want outsiders pouring into Angkor Wat. "We want visitors to regard [a visit to Angkor Wat] as a pilgrimage," says one Cambodian. "We don't want 20,000 tourists a day." As that person points out, Angkor Wat was not built as a museum but as a sacred place for the people of Cambodia.

QUESTIONS
1. What beliefs inspired the building of Angkor Wat?
2. Name two important features of Angkor Wat.
3. Why did the Khmer leave Angkor Wat?
4. What damage has Angkor Wat suffered?
5. What decision must Cambodians make about the future of Angkor Wat?

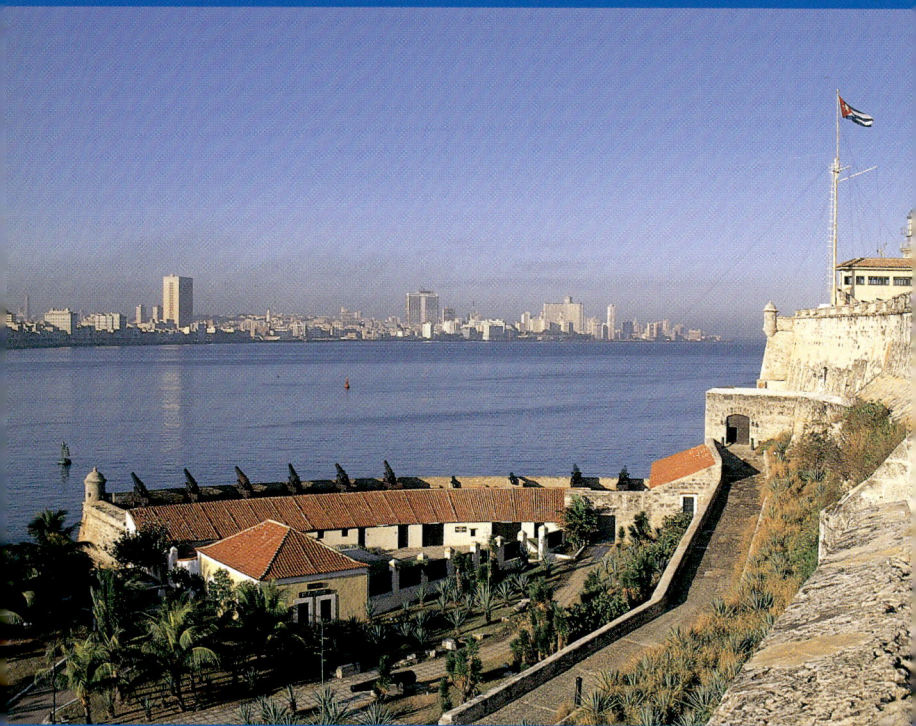

Remedios Diaz-Oliver was born in Cuba, an island south of Florida. When cuban life worsened under Fidel Castro, Diaz-Oliver fled to the United States.

Business Leader REMEDIOS DIAZ-OLIVER

How did Remedios Diaz-Oliver
[rĕ mĕ′dyōs dē′äs ō lē vĕr′]
go from prisoner to top business leader?

1 Life was easy at first for Remedios Diaz-Oliver. Her father was a rich hotel owner in Cuba. When she was a young girl, Diaz-Oliver went with her father on business trips to the United States and to Spain. So she saw countries and cultures other than her own.

2 Diaz-Oliver's native tongue, of course, was Spanish. But she also learned to speak English, French, and Italian. She went to good schools and finished high school a year early. She earned a doctorate[1] [dŏk′tər ĭt] in education from the University of Havana. Her plan was to become a teacher.

---
[1] doctorate: the highest university degree

Trouble in Cuba

3 In 1959, Fidel Castro [fē dĕl′ kăs′trō] came to power in Cuba. He promised Cubans a better life but gave them a communist dictatorship.[2]

4 Diaz-Oliver's family backed Castro because the old regime[3] [rā zhēm′] had been corrupt. The family had hoped for better times under Castro, an old family friend. Instead, Castro began to take away people's rights. In 1960, Castro saw Diaz-Oliver. He remembered her from when she was a child. "How are you?" Castro asked.

5 "Surprised," she answered, "that you didn't keep your promises."

6 Perhaps Castro did not jail Diaz-Oliver then because she was pregnant. But in 1961, Castro had her arrested and jailed for a short time. Diaz-Oliver had protested when Castro had people's mail checked. Castro feared an overthrow of his government. So he had inspectors check letters to Cuba for word of any plans for a revolt. When Diaz-Oliver was freed, she fled to the United States with her husband and daughter.

Starting Over

7 Now a refugee[4] [rĕf yōō jē′], Diaz-Oliver was nearly broke and in need of work. She was a

---

[2] dictatorship: a government run by one ruler with complete control

[3] regime: a government in power

[4] refugee: a person who flees to another country for safety

teacher but was not certified[5] to teach in the United States.

8   She found a job with Emmer Glass, a firm that sold containers. Diaz-Oliver earned only $10 a day, but she soon saw a chance to better herself. She knew that Emmer Glass wanted to attract buyers from Cuba and other parts of Latin America. Diaz-Oliver's Spanish language skills would be useful to the company.

9   She began to study the container business. She wanted to know all there was to know. She read every book and catalog she could find. Soon she was an expert in the field.

10   Within a year, Diaz-Oliver got a big promotion.[6] Emmer Glass put her in charge of all foreign sales. She sold huge numbers of containers to Central America. Within 10 years, Emmer Glass ranked first among firms that sold containers to places in Central America. Diaz-Oliver's hard work earned her the "E" Award. The "E" stands for Excellence in Export.[7] Diaz-Oliver received the award from the president of the United States. She was the first Hispanic business leader—male or female—to win this prize.

---

[5] certified: licensed
[6] promotion: a move up in position or rank
[7] export: the business of sending something overseas, especially to sell in another country

Dealing with Prejudice

11   One key to Diaz-Oliver's success was staying cool under pressure. Some people did not want to do business with her because she was Hispanic. Others wouldn't deal with her because she was female. But she never showed anger. Instead, she responded calmly with good humor and did her job well.

12   One male buyer who got Diaz-Oliver on the phone thought she was a secretary. He asked to talk to the boss. Diaz-Oliver told him that she *was* the boss. "I will never do business with a woman," he said. "And I will never do business with a Cuban." She calmly told him that he didn't have to and had him speak with a co-worker.

13   A year later, the man came crawling back. He needed Diaz-Oliver to help him out of a tight spot. She came through for him, and she did it without hard feelings. Soon the two became friends. The client even invited Diaz-Oliver to attend his son's wedding. (The son was marrying a Cuban woman!) The man also recommended her to other clients. Diaz-Oliver once said, "You can't get anything accomplished with anger. Everyone discriminates."[8]

---

[8] discriminate: to treat some people worse (or better) than others without any fair or proper reason

Her Own Company

14 In 1976, Diaz-Oliver took a big step. She and her husband started their own firm, a supplier of glass and plastic bottles. Diaz-Oliver's knowledge and years in the business helped to make it a success. In just one year, the company made close to a million dollars in sales. In 1991, sales reached $90 million. That same year, Diaz-Oliver started a family business with her husband and two children.

15 She was asked how she became so successful. Diaz-Oliver said, "I don't think [my success] is about being a woman or a minority as much as it is going into the boardroom with the same knowledge as men." ◆

QUESTIONS

1. Why did the future look bright for Diaz-Oliver as a young girl?
2. Why was she thrown in jail?
3. How did she go from a $10-a-day job to that of a top business leader?
4. How did she handle discrimination?

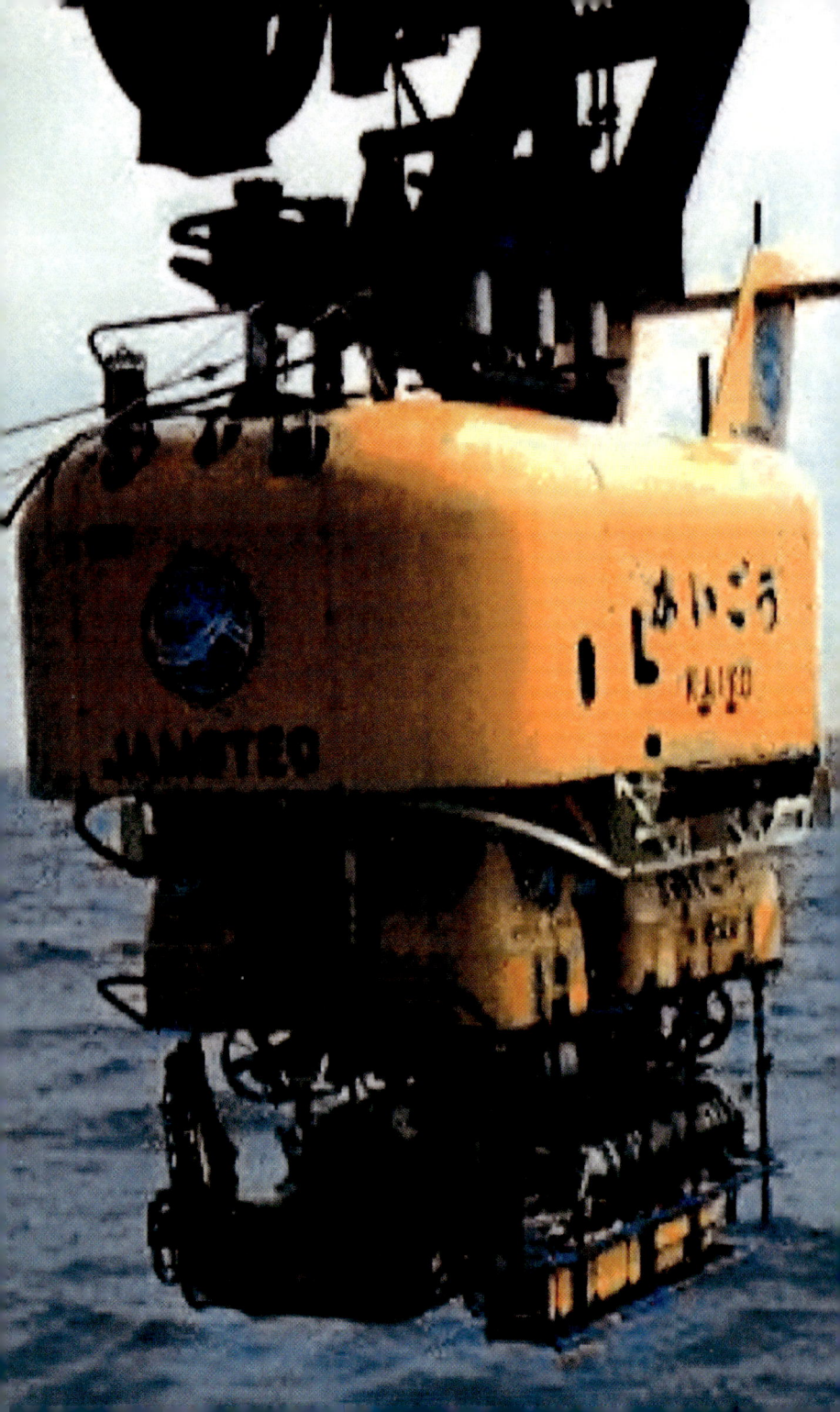

Exploring the Last Frontier

What are the risks and rewards of exploring the ocean's depths?

1 Humans have climbed Mount Everest. They have crossed the Sahara Desert and even lived at the South Pole. But one place on Earth that remains unconquered is the floor of the ocean. Scientists know more about the Moon and Mars than they do about the bottom of the sea. The ocean abyss[1] [ə bĭs′] is truly Earth's last great frontier.

Deep, Very Deep

2 Just how deep is the ocean? On average, it is about 2.3 miles deep. But some places are much deeper than that. The Mariana Trench lies under the Pacific Ocean. It is a 1,584-mile-long crevasse [krĭ văs′], or deep crack, in the ocean floor. The

---

[1] abyss: something so deep that it seems to have no bottom

In 1995, Japan sent *Kaiko*, an underwater vehicle run by remote control, to explore the deepest part of the ocean. The pictures *Kaiko* brought back proved that some creatures can live even seven miles under the sea.

deepest part of the trench is called Challenger Deep. At more than 36,000 feet down, it is the deepest spot in the world. That's a depth of nearly seven miles—a mile and a half deeper than Mount Everest is high.

3   People once thought that the ocean floor was flat and dull. Now they know better than that: the bottom of the ocean is much rougher than dry land. It has huge canyons, some of which are deep enough and large enough to hide the Rocky Mountains. The ocean floor also has its own mountain ranges. They are massive; one such range is more than 31,000 miles long. Circling the globe, it makes its way through all four of the world's oceans.

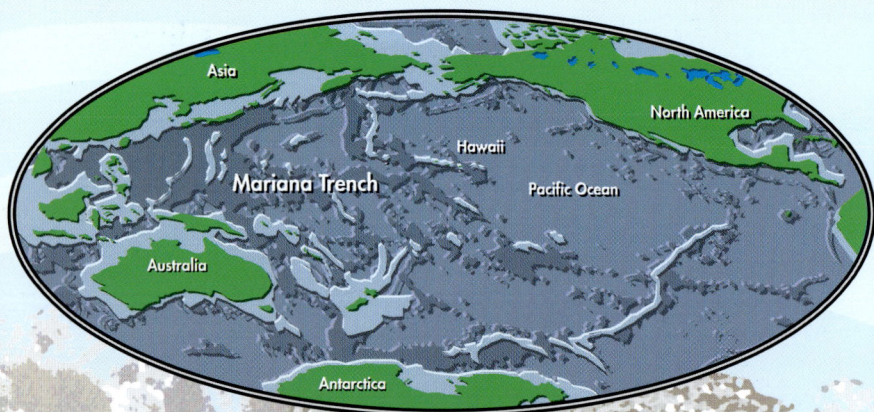

Far from being a flat plain, the ocean floor is rough and has many high and low features: divers can enter an underwater world of mountains and deep canyons. The deepest place is a long crack called the Mariana Trench, nearly seven miles beneath the Pacific Ocean.

Facing the Limits

4   The ocean has kept its secrets well. In some ways, it is harder to explore the seas than to explore outer space. One reason is that a human being, without help, can dive down only about ten feet. Beyond that depth, pressure starts to build on the lungs and inner ear. In any case, even the best diver can't hold his or her breath longer than two or three minutes.

5   Today, of course, divers can go much deeper than ever before. Those who use scuba gear can go down more than 100 feet. Scuba divers rarely go below 150 feet, though, for there is too much pressure. Coming back up can also be a problem. The change in pressure can cause the bends.[2] A bad case can be fatal. Wearing a pressurized suit, however, a diver can go down about 1,400 feet. From that point to the deepest part of the ocean is still a long distance.

The *Trieste*

6   In 1960, Donald Walsh and Jacques Piccard [zhäk pē kär′] climbed into a small metal sphere. It was a bathyscaphe [băth′ĭ skăf]— a watertight cabin used for deep-sea diving. Named the *Trieste* [trē ĕst′], the cabin carried nothing but the two men. It had no cameras to

---

[2] the bends: an illness caused by gas bubbles in the bloodstream

take pictures or arms to collect objects. The question was simple: could the two men go to the bottom of the Mariana Trench and come back alive?

7   It took Walsh and Piccard an hour and a half to descend 10,000 feet. Two hours later, they had gone down 32,000 feet. Pressure at this depth was immense—almost 14,000 pounds per square inch. After another hour, Walsh and Piccard were just 250 feet from the bottom of the ocean. Very slowly, they dropped down to the ocean floor. They had made it.

How Deep is Deep Enough?

8   That event happened a long time ago. Science has made great progress since then. Yet no one has ever duplicated[3] Walsh's and Piccard's feat. No other vehicle operated by humans has even come close. The reason is money—the trips are too costly.

9   In addition, some people aren't sure that exploring the ocean is worth the effort. Robert Ballard is the scientist who found the wreck of the *Titanic*. "I believe that the deep sea has very little to offer," he says. "I don't see the future there."

10   Jean Jarry [zhăn zhä rē], a top French ocean scientist, agrees. He doesn't feel that people

---

[3] duplicate: to repeat

should go below 20,000 feet. Only about 3 percent of the ocean is deeper than that. "To go beyond [20,000 feet] is not very interesting and is very expensive," Jarry says.

11   Others, however, disagree. Greg Stone, of the New England Aquarium, wants to go all the way down. He says, "We won't know what [the ocean floor] holds until we've been there."

12   The Japanese also want to explore the ocean abyss. In 1995, they sent an unmanned probe[4] named *Kaiko* [kī′ kō] to the bottom of Challenger Deep. *Kaiko* sent back pictures of things that were hard to believe—animals able to live at that depth. *Kaiko* saw a sea slug, a worm, and a shrimp. When they were there, Walsh and Piccard said they had seen a fish, but at the time few people believed them. Most people felt that nothing could live at such a depth. But now there is information that such life is possible.

With Humans or Without?

13   Should humans explore the abyss? Or should the work be left to remotely-controlled probes like *Kaiko*? Some scientists think that only humans can do the job correctly, fixing problems on the spot. They also say that nothing substitutes for

---

[4] probe: a machine used to explore an unknown area

being there in person. "Being able to see the deep-sea environment with your own eyes is vital," says one scientist.

14   Other scientists think that robots like *Kaiko* can do the job just as well. They argue that these unmanned probes are much cheaper to build. And, without risk to human life, robots are able to stay underwater a long time. Humans, meanwhile, can stay on land and watch a video screen to see what the robot sees.

Riches of the Deep

15   The deep sea contains great wealth. The ocean floor has untold amounts of iron, nickel, copper, and cobalt.[5] As scientists have found, many living things exist far beneath the waves. These include plants, fish, and bacteria. Yet, little is known about them. Like the plants in a rain forest, underwater life may hold the key to new miracle drugs. Scientists might not know the secrets of the deep today, but they know where to go to learn them.

---

[5] cobalt: a hard, metallic substance that looks like nickel and iron

QUESTIONS

1. What limits do human divers face?
2. Where did the *Trieste* go?
3. Why hasn't anyone gone to the bottom of the Mariana Trench since 1960?
4. Why do scientists use robots to explore the deep sea?
5. What riches are in the deep sea?

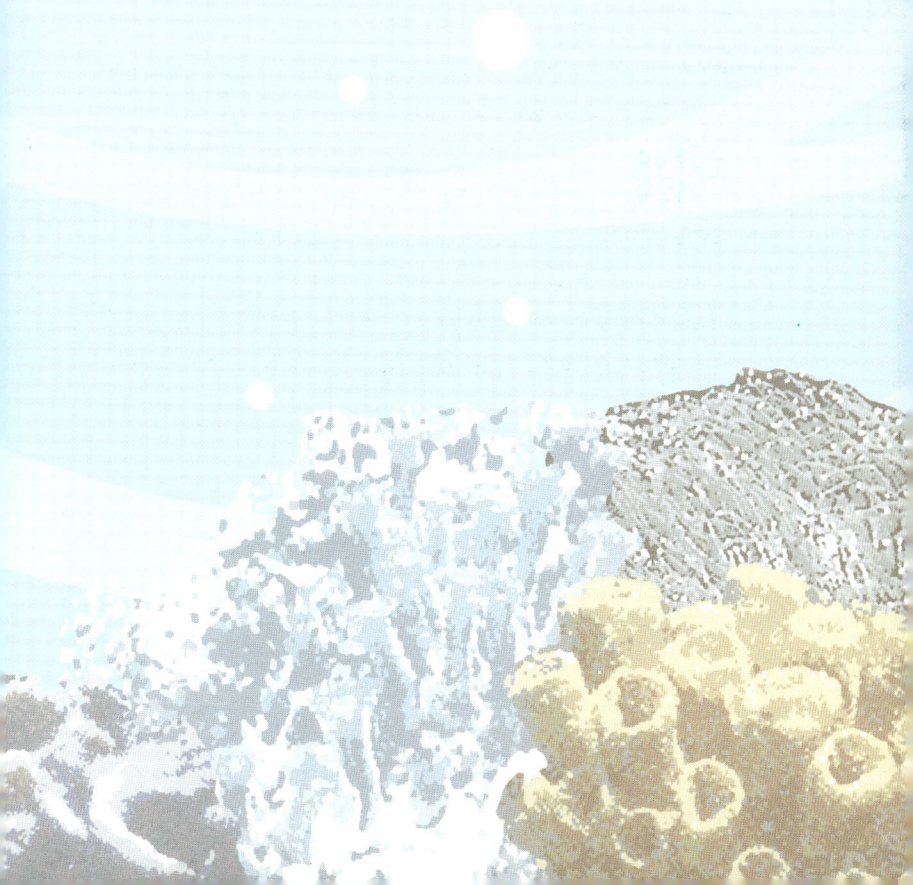

PHOTO CREDITS

Cover Image Bank. **vi** Dean Conger/National Geographic Image Collection. **4** Dean Conger/National Geographic Image Collection **8** Robert Baker. **11** Robert Baker. **13** UP/Wide World. **16** Reuters/Corbis-Bettmann. **19** Corbis-Bettmann. **20** Agence France Presse/Corbis-Bettmann. **22** Reuters/Corbis-Bettmann. **24** Corbis-Bettmann. **27** UPI/Corbis-Bettmann. **28** UPI/Corbis-Bettmann. **31** UPI/Corbis-Bettmann. **34** Darrell Gullin/Tony Stone. **36** Robert Frerck/Tony Stone. **38** Dick Durrance © National Geographic Society. **42** UPI/Corbis Bettmann. **45** Corbis-Bettmann. **48** NTC/Contemporary Books. **50** Philadelphia Museum of Art: Gift of Dr. and Mrs. Matthew T. Moore. **52** The Phillips Collection. **55** Albright-Knox Art Gallery, Buffalo, New York. **57** Philadelphia Museum of Art: Given by Robert Carlen. **58** © 1994, The Art Institute of Chicago, All Rights Reserved. **60** Schwart/Image Bank **62** J. Carmichael, Jr./Image Bank. **66** P. Goetgheluck/Image Bank. **68** Carlos Navajas/Image Bank. **73** Andrea Pistolesi/ Image Bank. **76** Chris Cheadle/Tony Stone. **82** Courtesy of JAMSTEC..

ILLUSTRATIONS

Mitch Lopata